T0095723

100 NATURAL FOODS

A Practical Guide to Health with
Traditional Chinese Medicine

A Modern Reader of
Compendium of Materia Medica

By Yang Li

Better Link Press

Editor's note: For your convenience, we have listed ingredient amounts in two measurement systems, printing both grams and ounces. Readers should feel free to modify the quantity of various ingredients according to their own preferences and dietary habits.

Copyright © 2019 by Shanghai Press and Publishing Development Co., Ltd.
Chinese edition © 2013 Chemical Industry Press

This book is edited and designed by the Editorial Committee of *Cultural China* series.

Text by Yang Li
Translation by Cao Jianxin
Design by Wang Wei

Copy Editors: Yang Xiaohe (Chinese), Gretchen Zampogna (English)
Editor: Cao Yue
Editorial Director: Zhang Yicong

Senior Consultants: Sun Yong, Wu Ying, Yang Xinci
Managing Director and Publisher: Wang Youbu

ISBN: 978-1-60220-160-6

Address any comments about *100 Natural Foods: A Practical Guide to Health with Traditional Chinese Medicine* to:

Better Link Press
99 Park Ave
New York, NY 10016
USA

or

Shanghai Press and Publishing Development Co., Ltd.
F 7 Donghu Road, Shanghai, China (200031)
Email: comments_betterlinkpress@hotmail.com

Printed in China by Shanghai Donnelley Printing Co., Ltd.

1   3   5   7   9   10   8   6   4   2

The material in this book is provided for informational purposes only and is not intended as medical advice. The information contained in this book should not be used to diagnose or treat any illness, disorder, disease or health problem. Always consult your physician or health care provider before beginning any treatment of any illness, disorder or injury. Use of this book, advice, and information contained in this book is at the sole choice and risk of the reader.

Quanjing provides the images on pages 30 and 188.

Contents

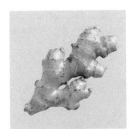
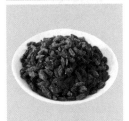
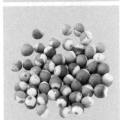
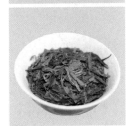

Fig.1 (From top to bottom)
ginger, Chinese wolfberries,
fox nuts and green tea leaves.

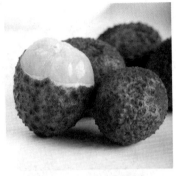

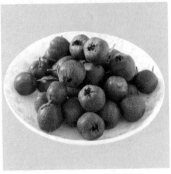

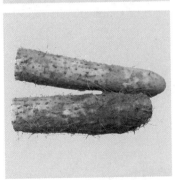

Fig. 2 (From top to bottom) lychees, hawthorn berries and yams.

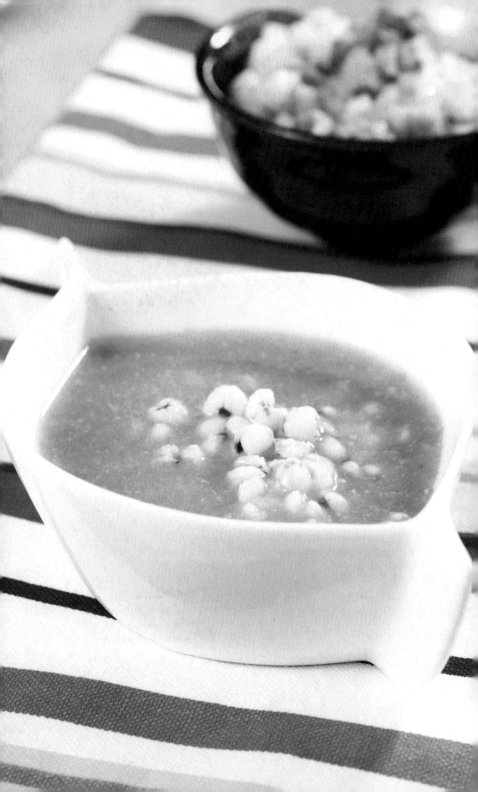

Introduction

It's common knowledge that every medicine has side effects. However, when people don't understand these side effects, they can often misuse drugs, resulting in many adverse consequences. Instead of emphasizing drug therapy, Traditional Chinese Medicine (TCM) has focused on using food for health preservation since ancient times. Most doctors in the past have advocated that "drug therapy is not as good as food therapy." It is better to have three carefully considered meals a day than to take medicine to prevent or cure illness. During the Ming Dynasty (1368–1644), great medical scientist and naturalist Li Shizhen (1518–1593) expressed this idea in the *Compendium of Materia Medica*. Today people are increasingly recognizing food therapy as the key to enhancing the human body's resistance.

In examining traditional health-preserving recipes, we will find that many common ingredients have unusual medicinal and health-preserving functions. Eating the right food at the right time is the best way to keep fit. Food therapy is not only more economical than drug therapy, but more importantly, the materials used in food therapy are natural, without side effects on the body.

Food ingredients are of great importance to human health in both ordinary times and after an illness. Although taking nutritional supplements after illness can be necessary due to physical weakness, there may be cases when one is too weak to be tonified. Eating nourishing food to build up one's body during healthy times can enhance one's health and reduce the incidence of disease. Of course, whether taking tonics in ordinary times or taking food therapy after illness, one should choose suitable food therapies based on one's physical conditions, symptoms and age.

These ideas are explored in the *Compendium of Materia Medica*, which is not only a medical work, but also a collection of healthy recipes. This TCM classic was also praised by Darwin (1809–1882) as the "oriental masterpiece in medicine." It contains 1,892 medicines and more than 11,000 prescriptions. The book divides medicines into three

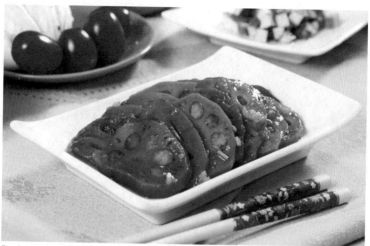

Fig. 3 Honeydew Sweet Lotus Root, see page 171 for the recipe.

types: mineral medicines, botanical medicines and animal medicines, each of which is divided into 16 classes and further divided into 60 categories, thus forming a sophisticated scientific classification system following the biological evolutionary laws from inorganic to organic, from simple to complex, and from low to high. The achievement of the *Compendium of Materia Medica* is that it's not only a masterpiece of pharmacy, but it also covers extensive topics and makes outstanding contributions to the fields of biology, chemistry, geology, astronomy, and more. It is also an encyclopedia and a masterpiece of ancient China's natural history.

Through personal practice and rigorous research, Li Shizhen detailed the name, origin, form, cultivation, collection, processing methods, preservation methods, medicinal properties, main indications, prescriptions and other aspects when explaining each drug, presenting detailed and scientific drug knowledge. In this medical classic, there are a great many food-based medicines derived from fruits, vegetables, grains, fish, nuts, drinks, etc., that people still eat today. Opening this ancient tome, you will find that Li Shizhen not only describes food, but also connects people and food naturally, telling readers what kind of food is useful to what kind of people and who should eat more, so that people can learn to choose food that is good for themselves and achieve the effect of food therapy in the broadest sense. Learning to use the food therapy in the *Compendium of Materia Medica* will help you better control your health. Therefore, this book explores the essence of the *Compendium of Materia Medica* by choosing nearly 100 kinds of food that can be seen everywhere in life, from the perspective of using ancient knowledge in a modern way, combining the dietary habits of contemporary people and the convenience of available ingredients. Note that some of the ingredients in this book are easy to find online, and others might be found only in specialty Asian markets. This book continues the wisdom of food therapy in the Traditional Chinese Medicine presented in the *Compendium of Materia Medica*, advocating health preservation and disease prevention by using the medicinal effects of pure natural foods.

Chapter One of this book explains the relationship among the properties, colors and tastes of different food and the internal organs of the human body, the laws of diet in each season and the methods of judging your own constitution in a refined and easy-to-understand way. Starting from Chapter Two, this book introduces nearly 100 kinds of food divided into eight major categories: grains, vegetables, fruits, meat, drinks, etc., with each category listed in a separate chapter, then comprehensively introduces the health effects of each food and presents rich dietary knowledge, guiding you to lasting health derived from natural foods.

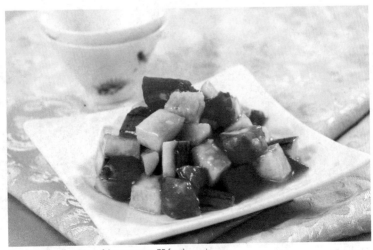

Fig. 4 Tomatoes and Loofahs, see page 75 for the recipe.

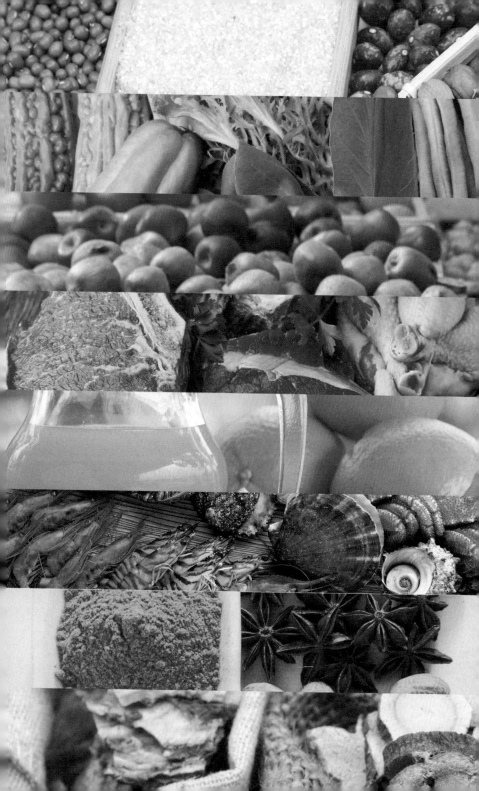

Chapter One
Choose the Right Food

With so many ingredients to choose from in daily life, are you ever confused when deciding which food is right for you? It might help to understand that the color and taste of each natural food ingredient have their own unique health effects and can nourish corresponding organs. For example, in terms of color, red food nourishes the heart and green food nourishes the liver; in terms of taste, sweet food nourishes the spleen, while salty food nourishes the kidneys. Food also has different properties. Some food can warm your body while some can help you clear your heat. You need to judge which food can help you according to your own constitution and physical conditions. In addition, the changing seasons also affect our bodies to different degrees. You should follow specific health preservation rules in each season to align your body with Mother Nature and maximize your health. Such knowledge of food therapy is detailed in the *Compendium of Materia Medica* and is applied through Traditional Chinese Medicine today.

This chapter will introduce the different health effects of five properties, colors and tastes of food, and explain how to reasonably follow the changing seasons with your diet. In addition, you can use the knowledge introduced in this chapter to start learning how to determine your own constitution and to apply scientific food therapy, thus achieving balance and health naturally at meals.

1. Five Properties of Food

The five properties of food relate to the human body's five reactions when food is eaten, which can be generally grouped into coldness, coolness, warmth, hotness and neutral. Knowing the five properties of food can allow you to have a better diet.

Five Properties	Health Effects	Recommended Food
Cold	Foods with cold properties have the effects of clearing heat, purging pathogenic fire, promoting the secretion of body fluids, relieving heat and detoxifying the body, and are suitable for people with excess of yang qi (yang vitality), a hot constitution or heat syndrome. The symptoms of excess of yang qi include acne on the face, dental ulcers, feeling hot all over the body, perspiring, flushing, having a dry mouth, having dry feces, being easily agitated or restless, and having a red tongue with a thin or thick yellow coating. The symptoms of a relatively hot body constitution include being easily agitated, irritated and annoyed, having a tendency to eat cold food or drink cold beverages—for example feeling the mouth is parched and the tongue scorched even when drinking water, having a flushed face, feeling hot all over the body and being sensitive to hot temperatures, and experiencing frequent constipation or dry feces, oliguria or yellow urine. The symptoms of heat syndrome include a dislike of warm things and a preference for cold things, feeling thirsty and being addicted to cold drinks, having a flushed face, being vexed and agitated, having thick, yellow phlegm and nasal mucus, experiencing hematemesis and bleeding from five-sense organs or subcutaneous tissue, having scanty, dark urine or dry feces, having red tongue or dry, yellow, coated tongue, etc.	Bitter melons, mung beans, tomatoes, bracken, bamboo shoots, lotus roots, water chestnuts, sugar cane, persimmons, mulberries, pears, kiwis, dragon fruits, melons, kelp, crabs, clams, field-snails, duck meat.
Cool	Foods with cool properties have the effect of clearing heat, promoting urination and	Millet, barley, wheat,

Five Properties	Health Effects	Recommended Food
Cool	detoxifying the body; these are suitable for people with yin deficiency, excess of yang qi, hot constitution or heat syndrome. The symptoms of yin deficiency include dizziness and tinnitus, insomnia and dreamful sleep, amnesia, soreness and weakness of the waist and knees, excess sexual desire, spermatorrhea, scanty menstruation, amenorrhea, or metrorrhagia and metrostaxis, emaciation, dry throat and mouth, hot flashes, dysphoria with a feverish sensation in the chest, palms and soles of the feet, night sweats, and a red tongue with little or no coating.	buckwheat, pearl barley, tofu, duck eggs, eggplant, white turnips, cucumbers, white gourds, loofahs, water bamboo, water spinach, seaweed, mung bean sprouts, spinach, amaranth, celery, oranges, watermelons, apples, rabbit meat.
Warm	Foods with warm properties have the effects of warming the spleen and stomach, dispelling cold and invigorating yang; they can also enhance physical power and strengthen the body. These are suitable for people with a relatively cold constitution, deficiency of yang or cold symptoms; they are also suitable for a warm supplement in autumn. The symptoms of a relatively cold body constitution include a tendency toward a plump and less muscular physique, an intolerance of cold temperatures, tendency to have cold limbs, a preference for hot food and drink, dispiritedness and a fat, tender, light-colored tongue. The symptoms of yang deficiency include intolerance of cold temperatures, cold limbs, a pale complexion, diarrhea with undigested food, dispiritedness, thin,	Glutinous rice, sorghum rice, goose eggs, Chinese chives, cumin, coriander, pumpkins, longans, papayas, pomegranates, dark plums, chestnuts, red dates, gingers, walnuts, almonds, chicken, beef, mutton, shrimp, sea cucumbers, garlic, onions, green onions.

Five Properties	Health Effects	Recommended Food
Warm	sloppy stool and clear, abundant urine. Cold symptoms are uncomfortable symptoms caused by a cold body constitution, such as an intolerance of cold temperature.	
Hot	Foods with hot properties have an obvious warming effect, which is more likely to produce warmth than food with warm properties, so these are suitable for people of cold constitution. The symptoms of a cold body constitution include pale complexion, light color of lips and mouth, tendency toward fatigue, fear of cold temperature and wind, cold limbs, preference for hot drinks and foods, frequent diarrhea, prolonged menstrual cycle, a light tongue color and a white coating on the tongue.	Chili, garlic sprouts, garlic bolts, lychees, trout.
Neutral	Foods with neutral properties have the effects of promoting the appetite, strengthening the spleen, strengthening the body and tonifying deficiency. People with different constitutions, cold, cool or heat syndromes can all eat such food. The cold, cool or heat syndromes are all kinds of symptoms caused by cold body constitution or hot body constitution.	Rice, corn, peanuts, soybeans, red beans, black beans, eggs, milk, potatoes, taro, lotus seeds, hazelnuts, fox nuts, mushrooms, white fungus, black fungus, Chinese cabbage, shepherd's purse, cabbage, carrots, plums, figs, grapes, pork, goose, yellow croaker, pomfret, black carp, crucian carp.

2. Five Colors of Food

Natural food can be classified into five categories according to their colors on the surface: green food, red food, yellow food, white food and black food. According to the Chinese medicine, the five internal organs of human body correspond to these different colors: red food nourishes the heart, green food nourishes the liver, yellow food nourishes the spleen, white food nourishes the lungs and black food nourishes the kidneys.

Five Colors	Corre-sponding Organs	Health Effects	Recommended Food
Red	Heart	Red food is rich in carotene, and along with other nutrients contained in red food, this helps enhance cell viability, improve the body's ability to prevent and cure colds, and promote blood circulation to remove blood stasis. Another advantage of red food lies in its rich natural iron content; for example, cherries and red dates are natural medicines for patients with anemia, and they can also be taken as nourishing food for women after menstrual blood loss.	Beef, mutton, pork liver, red peppers, red sweet peppers, red amaranth, red perilla, hawthorn berries, tomatoes, watermelon, red dates, persimmons, strawberries, cherries, plums, purple yams, red beans, "red heart" sweet potatoes, red wine.
Green	Liver	Most green foods are vegetables, and they are rich in vitamin C. High vitamin C intake helps enhance immunity and prevent diseases. For those who have high work tension, spend a lot of time in computer operation, or who smoke, higher vitamin C intake is recommended; green food also provides a variety of vitamins and dietary fiber, as well as promotes toxin expulsion and skin moisturization.	Spinach, cabbage mustard, rapeseed greens, broccoli, Chinese chives, loofahs, bitter gourds, green soybeans, peas, asparagus, muskmelons, guavas, kiwis.

Five Colors	Corresponding Organs	Health Effects	Recommended Food
Yellow	Spleen	The biggest advantage of yellow food is that it's rich in vitamins A and D. Vitamin A helps protect the gastric mucosa and prevent diseases such as stomach ulcers and gastritis; vitamin D promotes calcium and phosphorus absorption, so yellow food's functions include toning up muscles and bones.	Pearl barley, oats, brown rice, peanuts, "yellow heart" sweet potatoes, pumpkins, daylilies, corn, hotbed chives, soybeans, lemons, pineapples, bananas, oranges, papayas, citrus, loquats, sugarcane, honey.
White	Lungs	White food has the effect of moistening the lungs, and it helps regulate eyesight and promote emotional stability. White food is quite beneficial to the patient with hypertension and heart disease.	Fish, rice, glutinous rice, yams, lotus seeds, flour, almonds, white gourds, bamboo shoots, water bamboo, lotus roots, milk, bean curd, soy milk, skin of tofu, egg whites, pears, lychees, coconuts, white fungus, white radishes, white sugar, lily bulbs.
Black	Kidneys	Black food is rich in amino acids and minerals, and its benefits include tonifying the kidneys, nourishing the blood and moisturizing the skin; it also has health-care functions such as skin protection, anti-aging, etc. For this reason, it is known as "life-extending food."	Black rice, black sesame, black fungus, black beans, seaweed, kelp, black-bone chicken, mushrooms, black dates, mulberries, preserved eggs, fermented soybeans, dark plums, soy sauce, sea cucumbers, cuttlefish.

3. Five Tastes of Food

The five tastes refer to bitter, sour, sweet, spicy and salty flavors of food. Besides these five tastes, there are bland taste and astringent taste; usually the bland taste is associated with sweet taste while the astringent taste is related to salty taste. Foods correspond to different meridians because they have different flavors: Sour corresponds to the liver, spicy corresponds to the lungs, bitter corresponds to the heart, salty corresponds to the kidneys and sweet corresponds to the spleen.

Five Tastes	Corre-sponding Internal Organs	Health Effects	Recommended Food
Bitter	Heart	The effects of bitter foods include eliminating internal heat and purging pathogenic fire, reducing anger and dysphoria, detoxification, diminishing inflammation, and invigorating the stomach and spleen. Bitter flavors also have anti-microbial and antiviral functions. However, too much bitter food can lead to dyspepsia.	Bitter gourds, bitter herbs, Chinese toon, ginkgo, dandelions, almonds, honeysuckle, tea leaves.
Sour	Liver	Sour flavors are astringent or capable of inducing astringency, and these foods help whet the appetite, tonify the spleen, enhance hepatic function and improve the absorption rate of calcium and phosphorus. However, eating too much sour food is detrimental to the muscles and bones.	Oranges, peaches, plums, lemons, olives, hawthorn berries, mangoes, grapes, grapefruits, tangerines, dark plums, apricots, vinegar.
Sweet	Spleen	Sweet-flavored foods tonify qi (vitality) and blood and strengthen the body, and are suitable for those with deficiency syndrome, such as qi deficiency, blood deficiency, yin deficiency and yang deficiency; sweet foods also help	Pearl barley, cucumbers, pumpkins, Chinese cabbage, sugar, spinach, sugarcane,

Five Tastes	Corresponding Internal Organs	Health Effects	Recommended Food
Sweet	Spleen	relieve muscle tension. However, overconsumption of sweet food brings a great risk of obesity. The symptoms of qi deficiency include poor health, pale complexion, shortness of breath, weak limbs, dizziness, sweating, fainting and a low voice. The symptoms of blood deficiency include pale or sallow complexion, light color of lips, tongue and nails, dizziness, palpitation and dreaminess, numb hands and feet, scanty menstruation, light menstrual color, opsomenorrhea or amenorrhea. The symptoms of yin deficiency include dizziness and tinnitus, insomnia and dreamful sleep, amnesia, soreness and weakness of waist and knees, excess sexual desire, spermatorrhea, scanty menstruation or amenorrhea, or metrorrhagia and metrostaxis, emaciated body, dry throat and mouth, hot flash, dysphoria with feverish sensation in the chest, palms and soles of the feet, night sweats, and a red tongue with little or no coating. The symptoms of yang deficiency include intolerance of cold temperatures, cold limbs, pale complexion, diarrhea with undigested food, dispiritedness, thin and sloppy stool, and clear, abundant urine. A doctor should make a professional diagnosis for these diseases.	apples, watermelons, red dates, honey, lily bulbs.

Five Tastes	Corresponding Internal Organs	Health Effects	Recommended Food
Spicy	Lungs	Spicy food disperses bad elements, promotes the circulation of qi and invigorates blood circulation. Eating spicy food promotes gastrointestinal peristalsis, enhances secretion of digestive juices, improves activity of amylase, and promotes blood circulation and metabolism. However, too much consumption may hurt body fluids and cause excessive internal heat.	Chilis, ginger, white part of green onion stalk, white radishes, purple perilla, fennel, cassia bark, spirits, medicinal liquors, black pepper.
Salty	Kidneys	Salty food is rich in mineral substances, and it helps eliminate phlegm, tonify the kidneys, soften and resolve hard lumps, and it can be used to cure diseases such as dry stool and so on. However, too much consumption may cause hypertension, atherosclerosis, and other problems.	Amaranth, kelp, seaweed, sea cucumbers, jellyfish, crabmeat, clams, snails, duck, pork, salt, soy sauce.

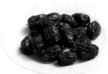
Fig. 5 Red dates.

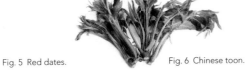
Fig. 6 Chinese toon.

4. How to Eat in Each Season

As the weather changes in spring, summer, autumn and winter, all things follow the natural order: They are born in spring, grow in summer, are harvested in autumn and stored in winter. We, who are living in nature, are affected by Mother Nature in every moment. Therefore, as Ming Dynasty famous medical scientist Zhang Jingyue (1563–1640) said, "For health preservation, people should nourish the liver in spring, nourish the heart and the spleen in summer, nourish the lungs in autumn and nourish the kidneys in winter." This is the truth.

Principles for Health Preservation in Spring

Spring is a season in which everything grows and refreshes. Food therapy generally uses neutral-property food in spring, along with acid, sweet and warm food, such as chicken, eggs, lean pork, and red dates. However, you should not eat only warm tonics, which could increase heat inside the body as temperatures rise with the season and impair the body's positive qi. In the early spring when the climate is still cold, the human body needs to consume a certain amount of energy to keep out the cold and maintain the basic body temperature. The nutrient composition during the early spring should mainly favor high-calorie food, and in addition to cereal products, soybeans, sesame seeds, peanuts, and walnuts can be used to replenish energy. In addition to diet, the following three points should be noted for health preservation in spring.

Focusing on nourishing the liver: The liver's health corresponds mainly to the spring. Nourishing the liver helps one avoid getting too tired in this season.

Preventing influenza: As the weather turns from cold to warm in the spring, warm-heat and toxic evil gradually begin to appear. People are prone to catching the flu during this time, but drinking plenty of water and eating more vegetables can help keep this illness at bay.

Doing more exercise: In the sunny spring, it is advisable to go outside, enjoy the flowers and climb mountains.

Principles for Health Preservation in Summer

Hot summer is the season when the body consumes the greatest amount of energy. The human body sweats more, and protein catabolism is enhanced, so people should increase protein intake in an appropriate amount. The daily intake of protein is ideally 100 to 120 grams, and more than half of this should be high-quality protein such as fish, lean meat, chicken, eggs, milk and bean products. High temperatures can increase the body's metabolism, and a lot of water, minerals and water-soluble vitamins such as vitamins C, B_1 and B_2 will be lost from sweat, thereby increasing the body's energy consumption and reducing its endurance and resistance. People should pay attention to timely replenishing water, minerals and vitamins, eating bitter foods, and eating more vegetables and fruits. In summer, people should pay attention to the following four points.

Focusing on resting to attain mental tranquility: One will feel cool if one's heart is peaceful. It is better not to become irritable in the hot weather, as it will cause the generation of internal heat.

Adjusting diet: In summer when yang qi is excessive and yin qi (yin vitality) is deficient, it is advisable to eat light and digestible food.

Nourishing body fluid: In summer, it is easy to lose body fluid due to excess sweating. It's important to stay hydrated and supplement lost minerals.

Preventing heatstroke: Avoid working or quick walking for a long time under the scorching sun. People can drink mung bean soup to relieve summer heat.

Principles for Health Preservation in Autumn

In autumn, the sky is clear and the air is crisp, but the climate is dry. As a result, the body is prone to fatigue. If you have unhealthy living habits, it is easy to have symptoms such as rapid heartbeat, hot body, chapped lips and restlessness. This is what people often call "getting excessive internal heat."

In autumn, people should eat more fresh food containing less oil but more vitamins and protein. Food rich in vitamins A, B, C, and E, such as carrots, lotus roots, pears, honey, sesame, and black fungus, can nourish the blood and relieve dryness, prevent chapped lips, and enhance disease resistance. Autumn is also a time to reduce the consumption of spicy food and increase the intake of sour food to nourish the liver and lungs. Some examples include pears, lotus seeds, lily bulbs, longans, red dates, chestnuts, white fungus, and water chestnuts. It's also advisable to eat some warm-property food such as beef and mutton to enrich the blood and enhance physical fitness. In addition to diet, the following four points should be noted for health preservation in autumn.

Nourishing the lung: With the main function of breathing, the lungs are connected to the throat and nose. Special attention should be paid to the lungs, as they are exposed to the irritations and influence of various external climates.

Preventing against dryness: In the autumn when the air is dry, people often have a fever, dry throat and nasal cavity, dry mouth and chapped lips etc., so hydration and moisturizing are important.

Staying cool in autumn for health: It is said that "one will not get sick if one wears warm in the spring and cool in the autumn." In autumn, one can also take cold water showers as appropriate.

Suitable for sports: As the climate cools in autumn, the season is perfect for outdoor sports like mountain climbing and jogging.

Principles for Health Preservation in Winter

Winter is a season when grass and trees wither and are frozen, insects hibernate, and all things in nature hide themselves. It is also the most suitable season for nourishment, which can regulate the metabolism of substances in the body, so that the energy converted from nutrients can be stored in the body to the maximum extent. This helps increase yang in the body and lay a good foundation for health in the coming year. In winter, you can choose to eat polished round-ground rice, corn, wheat, soybeans, peas, tangerines, pineapples, longans (fig.7), garlic, mutton, beef, chicken, fish, shrimp, etc., to increase the body's cold and disease resistance. In addition to food therapy, pay attention to the following three points for health preservation in winter.

Nourishing the kidney: Nourishment of the kidney in winter should be centered around the "water," with the nourishment of kidney water as the key.

Keeping warm and avoiding the cold and cool: Use warming methods to dispel pathogenic cold.

Eating tonics on the winter solstice: Winter is a great season to keep fit by eating tonics, as they can enhance physical fitness and improve disease resistance. One should choose tonics according to their own constitution and weakness of the inner organs. For example, if one is weak in the lungs, then foods and medicine that nourish the lungs are a good choice. Taking these nourishing foods in winter can have a more outstanding effect than in other seasons.

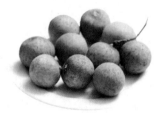

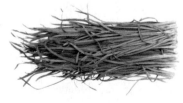

Fig. 7 Longans.

Fig. 8 Chinese leeks.

5. What to Eat for Different Constitutions

Some people are optimistic by nature, but some are always depressed; some are afraid of the cold and some are fearful of heat—this is due to different types of constitution. There are nine kinds of constitutions according to Chinese medicine: neutral type, qi deficient type, yang deficient type, yin deficient type, phlegm and dampness type, damp-heat type, blood stasis type, qi stagnation type, and special constitution type. Most people are marked by two or more than two complex temperaments. Choosing the most suitable foods according to different constitutions is a fundamental key to health care.

Neutral Type

Features: glowing complexion, energetic nature, tendency toward good sleep, and strong resistance to illness as manifestations of good health.

The dietary principle: Diet should be brought under control, maintaining a reasonable variety of foods, without too much of any particular food and with proper intake of quantity, as well as avoiding foods that are too cold, too hot or unclean; also decreasing intake of oily and spicy food.

Qi Deficient Type

Features: low and weak voice, fatigue from time to time, low spirits, easy sweating, poor resistance, vulnerability to the cold and difficulty recovering from illness.

The dietary principle: Food beneficial to qi and spleen should be added in an appropriate amount, such as yams, glutinous rice, millet, chicken, mushrooms, red dates, honey, sugar, and beef, etc. Turnip and water convolvulus should be avoided since they are detrimental to qi. In addition, it is a taboo to have raw and cold foods such as cold drinks, beer and icy watermelon, as well as oily and spicy foods.

Yang Deficient Type

Features: sensitivity to low temperatures, cold limbs, addiction to hot drinks and food, tender, fat and light-colored tongue, as well as a series of metabolic diseases such as obesity and disorder of glycolipid metabolism.

The dietary principle: Eat more foods with warm and hot properties with the functions of warming yang and dispelling cold, such as lychees, longans, cashews, ginger, Chinese leeks (fig. 8), peppers, beef etc. Eat less food with cool or cold properties, such as turnips, bean curd, bitter gourds, water chestnuts, watermelon, green beans, kelp or crab, etc. Especially avoid food directly taken out of the refrigerator.

Yin Deficient Type

Features: excessive internal heat, unknown heat and sweating in the palms and soles of the feet, tendency toward emotional upheaval and short sleep duration, and vulnerability to the contraction of TB, insomnia and tumors, etc.

The dietary principle: It is advisable to eat sweet and cool food that nourishes yin and promotes the secretion of body fluid, but in an appropriate amount so as not to harm the spleen and stomach. Food of this kind includes wheat, rice, millet, corn, buckwheat, black sesame, duck meat, duck eggs, water chestnuts, soft-shelled turtle, white fungus, black fungus, white cabbage, tomatoes, spinach, cucumbers, bitter gourds, loofahs, laver, grapes, pears, kiwis, grapefruits and watermelons. People should be cautious while eating spicy food, fried food and food with very high sugar and fat content, which will harm yin, produce internal heat and sputum, and result in aggravation of yin deficiency.

Phlegm and Dampness Type

Features: tendency to become overweight, dislike of drinking water, poor adaptability to damp environments, and vulnerability to the contraction of diabetes, obesity, fat liver and irregular menstruation, etc.

The dietary principle: It is advisable to eat more food rich in protein, fresh vegetables and fruits, whereas it is taboo to eat foods with lots of fat and sugar that produce high calories. In addition, avoid eating sweet food in the evening or before going to bed. Avoid eating cold and raw food as well as mutton and longans, which produce internal heat and increase dampness.

Damp-Heat Type

Features: oily face, bitter taste and dryness in mouth, stagnant discharge of excrement or dry excrement, vulnerability to the contraction of testis dampness, increase of leucorrhea, difficulty in adapting to damp or hot environments, and vulnerability to the contraction of skin disease, liver disease, gallbladder disease and diseases of the urogenital system.

The dietary principle: Eat more vegetables and fruits with high protein content. Eat less high-calorie, high-fat or high-cholesterol food, such as sweet food, fat meat and inner organs of animals, etc. Eat less sweet, warm-property, greasy, barbecued and fried food.

Blood Stasis Type

Features: dull complexion, precipitated pigments and ecchymosis, dark lips, dark tongue with petechiae, thick, dark and purplish veins under the tongue, forgetfulness, prone to agitation, tendency to get tumors and those diseases with pain as the main symptom.

   The dietary principle: Diet should be diversified, rather than restricted to particular kinds of food. Often eat vegetables and fruits such as carrots, coriander, shepherd's purses, ginger and tangerines, which serve to smooth qi and invigorate blood circulation. Avoid eating cold and raw food, which can cause blood condensation due to the cold and blocked blood circulation. Cold and raw food includes various kinds of cold drinks, salad, crab, river snails, pears, watermelons, cucumbers, grapefruits and water chestnuts (fig. 9).

Qi Stagnation Type

Features: introverted personality, poor adaptability to mental stimulation, dislike of cloudy or rainy weather, predisposition to depression, chronic gastritis, chronic sore throat, dysmenorrhoea, migraine and cyclomastopathy.

   The dietary principle: It is advisable to have a diet with low fat and high fiber to smooth the liver and regulate qi while promoting blood circulation. People are advised to eat more cereals, beans, and fresh vegetables and fruits while avoiding high-fat food, and eat less salty, spicy, sour and astringent foods such as preserved vegetables, pomegranates, sour-dates, plums and lemons, etc.

Special Constitution Type

Features: poor adaptability to the outer environment, susceptibility to the contraction of asthma, urticaria, hay fever and allergy to drugs, etc.

   The dietary principle: Pay attention to the balance of nutrition, with more intake of milk, fresh-water fish, bean products, and fresh vegetables and fruits in proper amounts. Try to avoid eating foods that can induce allergies such as sea fish, shrimps and crabs, as well as food with additives such as preserved fruit and candies. In addition, try to avoid alcoholic drinks and food that is too raw, cold, sour, salty or greasy.

Fig. 9 Water chestnuts.

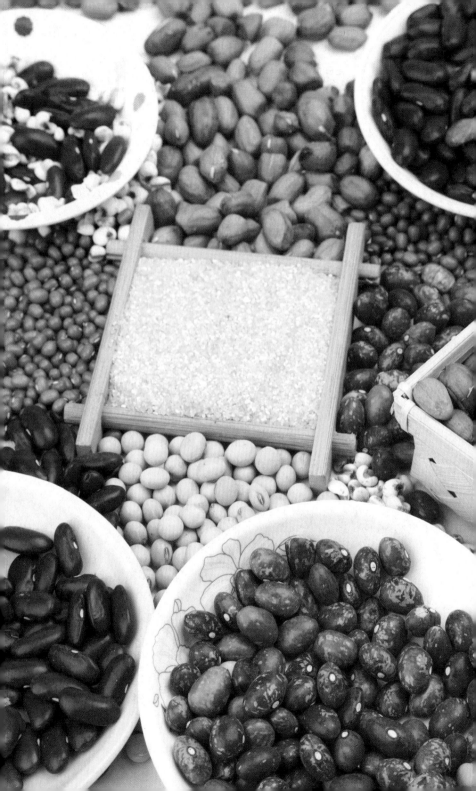

Chapter Two
Grains

Grains are an essential food for human beings. They are inexpensive and have a high digestibility and absorption rate, making them the most economical source of nutrition. Grains contain many beneficial ingredients and have many advantages that cannot be replaced by medicine.

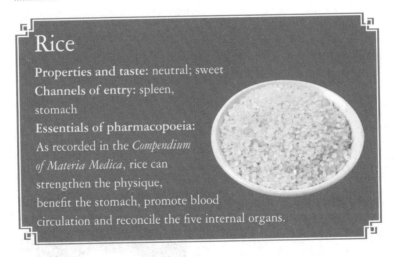

Rice

Properties and taste: neutral; sweet
Channels of entry: spleen, stomach
Essentials of pharmacopoeia:
As recorded in the *Compendium of Materia Medica*, rice can strengthen the physique, benefit the stomach, promote blood circulation and reconcile the five internal organs.

Health Effects
Preventing arteriosclerosis: Rice can provide necessary nutrients and energy for the body, and its rich dietary fiber can excrete bile in the intestines from the body, promote digestion and prevent arteriosclerosis.

Nourishing the skin and strengthening the body: Rice has the effects of tonifying qi, reinforcing the spleen, nourishing the stomach, benefiting the spirit and strengthening the mind, reconciling the five internal organs, promoting blood circulation, improving ear and eye functions, reducing irritability, quenching thirst and stopping diarrhea. Eating more rice can strengthen the body and improve the facial complexion.

Points of Attention for Different People

Suitable for babies: Rice soup can promote the absorption of nutrients in milk.

Suitable for elderly people: Rice soup can strengthen the functions of the spleen and stomach and enhance gastric motility.

Not suitable for people with diabetes: The rice gruel has a high blood sugar production index.

Food Compatibility and Incompatibility

Suitable: rice + mung beans = increases the utilization rate of the nutritional ingredients of rice

Suitable: rice + black rice = stimulates and improves the appetite

Avoid: rice + honey = tends to cause stomachache

Cooking Tip

When making rice gruel, do not use alkali, which will destroy the vitamin B_1 in rice. Braise rice instead of steaming after boiling and straining rice as the latter will lose a lot of vitamins.

Healthy Recipe

Rice and Sea Cucumber Porridge

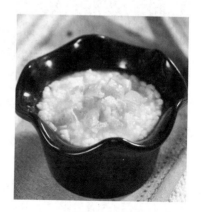

Ingredients: 100 g (3.5 oz) rice, two prepared sea cucumbers, 500 g (18 oz) water

Preparation: ❶Wash rice clean, wash the prepared sea cucumbers and cut them into small pieces. ❷Put rice and sea cucumbers into a pot, add water and cook them into porridge.

Corn

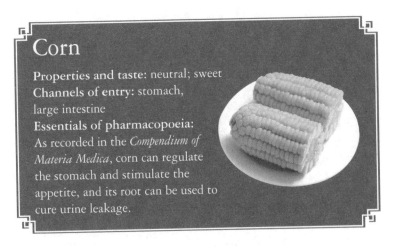

Properties and taste: neutral; sweet
Channels of entry: stomach, large intestine
Essentials of pharmacopoeia:
As recorded in the *Compendium of Materia Medica*, corn can regulate the stomach and stimulate the appetite, and its root can be used to cure urine leakage.

Health Effects

Nourishing the brain and anti-aging: Corn is rich in vitamin E, lecithin and glutamate, and it invigorates the brain and provides an antiaging effect.

Preventing cancer: Corn is rich in elements such as magnesium and selenium, which inhibit tumor growth.

Bringing down blood pressure and reducing blood glucose: The stigma of corn is rich in potassium nitrate, vitamin K, sitosterol, stigmasterol and a volatile alkaloid. Its functions include promoting urination, reducing hypertension, blood glucose and hemostasis, and promoting the flow of bile.

Points of Attention for Different People

Suitable for elderly people: Eating corn can protect the eyes from aging.

Suitable for patients with diabetes: The corn's dietary fiber absorbs glucose to reduce blood glucose concentration.

Not suitable for patients with enuresis: Corn can aggravate this disease.

Food Compatibility and Incompatibility

Suitable: corn + eggs = reduces the absorption of cholesterol

Suitable: corn + pine nuts = prevents heart disease, helps prevent cancer and increases resistance to cancer

Suitable: corn + pigeon meat = prevents neurasthenia

Cooking Tip

The nicotinic acid in corn can effectively prevent and cure skin diseases, but it isn't easily absorbed by the human body. Adding some alkali to corn during cooking helps break nicotinic acid into elements that can be more easily absorbed by the body.

Healthy Recipes

Corn Grit Porridge

Ingredients: 100 g (3.5 oz) corn, 50 g (2 oz) millet, 3 g (0.1 oz) rock candy

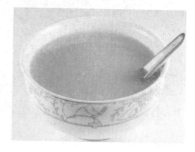

Preparation: ❶Wash the corn grit and millet. ❷Bring a pot of water to a boil, and boil clean corn grit for 10 minutes; then add the millet to the pot. ❸When the porridge is well-cooked and thick, add the rock candy.

Tip: Cooking the porridge with hot water rather than cold not only saves time, but also prevents burning the bottom of the pot.

Pine Nuts and Corn

Ingredients: 300 g (10.5 oz) corn kernels, 50 g (2 oz) pine nuts, 20 g (1 oz) green peppers, 15 g (0.5 oz) red peppers, 10 g (0.4 oz) each chopped green onion and white sugar, 4 g (0.1 oz) salt, 2 g (0.1 oz) each monosodium glutamate and sesame oil

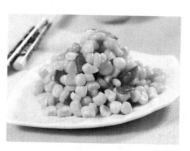

Preparation: ❶Wash green and red peppers, remove their pedicles and seeds, and dice them; put the corn into boiling water and boil until it is 80 percent cooked and chewable; get the corn out and drain well. ❷Heat some oil in a pan and add the pine nuts, fry until they turn light yellow, and dish it up. ❸Heat some more oil in the pan; put the chopped green onion into the pan and fry until fragrant; add diced red and green peppers and corn kernels to the pan and stir-fry them until they are cooked; season the dish with salt, monosodium glutamate, white sugar and sesame oil. Dish it up and sprinkle with some pine nuts to serve.

Millet

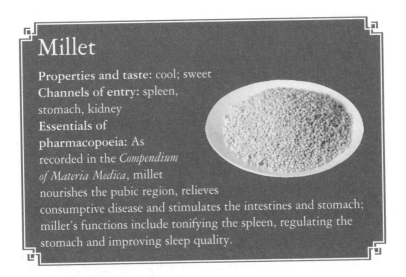

Properties and taste: cool; sweet
Channels of entry: spleen, stomach, kidney
Essentials of pharmacopoeia: As recorded in the *Compendium of Materia Medica*, millet nourishes the pubic region, relieves consumptive disease and stimulates the intestines and stomach; millet's functions include tonifying the spleen, regulating the stomach and improving sleep quality.

Health Effects

Regulating stomach function and improving sleep quality:
The tryptophan in millet nourishes the stomach and improves sleep quality; note that tryptophan can only be obtained from food. The carbohydrates in millet relieve symptoms such as mental stress, excessive pressure, fatigue and weakness.

Treating yin deficiency and nourishing blood: "Rice bran oil," a layer of sticky film-like ointment floating on the surface of millet congee, can regulate deficiency-cold body. After giving birth, the mother can nourish her body by eating millet congee.

Tonifying the spleen and helping digestion: The rice crust from the cooked millet is known as "golden powder," and it nourishes qi and tonifies the spleen, removes food retention and cures diarrhea. It can be taken as a dietary therapy for chronic diarrhea due to spleen deficiency, stomachache due to dyspepsia, and for children with dyspepsia.

Points of Attention for Different People

Suitable for parturients: The porridge is ideal food for women when they are recovering from postpartum weakness.

Suitable for patients with hypertension and skin disease:
Millet can help prevent hypertension and skin diseases.

Food Compatibility and Incompatibility

Suitable: millet + soybeans = improves the utilization rate of protein

Suitable: millet + longans = enriches the blood, nourishes the skin, soothes the nerves and improves brain health

Suitable: millet + carrots = protects the eyes and nourishes the skin

Avoid: millet + vinegar = damages the carotenoid millet contains

Cooking Tip

Do not cook millet with cold tap water, because the chlorine in the water will destroy vitamin B_1 in the process of boiling, which results in the loss of nutrients. Wash millet gently to avoid losing the grain's external layer and its rich nutrient content.

Healthy Recipe
Millet and Red Dates Porridge

Ingredients: 100 g (3.5 oz) millet, 30 g (1 oz) red dates (dried), 15 g (0.5 oz) red beans, 10 g (0.4 oz) brown sugar, 500 g (18 oz) water

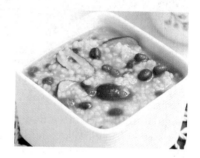

Preparation: ❶Wash the red beans and soak them for four hours; wash the millet; wash the red dates and core them, and then soak them for half an hour. ❷Bring a pot of water to a boil, then add some red beans and boil until they are half-cooked; add the clean millet and cored dates and simmer until thoroughly cooked; stir some brown sugar into the porridge to serve.

Black Rice

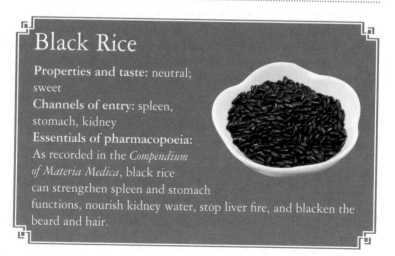

Properties and taste: neutral; sweet

Channels of entry: spleen, stomach, kidney

Essentials of pharmacopoeia: As recorded in the *Compendium of Materia Medica*, black rice can strengthen spleen and stomach functions, nourish kidney water, stop liver fire, and blacken the beard and hair.

Health Effects

Enriching the blood and improving eyesight: As a good nourishing product, black rice can sustain yin and tonify the kidneys and stomach, warm the liver, improve eyesight and promote blood circulation. It has good therapeutic effects on dizziness, anemia, gray hair and eye disease.

Preventing cancer: The trace element selenium contained in black rice has anti-cancer effects. Black rice is also rich in minerals such as manganese, zinc and iron, as well as vitamin C, chlorophyll, anthocyanin, carotene and other beneficial components.

Points of Attention for Different People

Suitable for women: Black rice blackens and protects hair, nourishes skin and maintains beauty.

Suitable for insomnia patients: Black rice improves sleep quality.

Suitable for anemia patients: With strong nourishing effect, black rice is known as "blood enriching rice."

Food Compatibility and Incompatibility

Suitable: black rice + rice = stimulates appetite, benefits the stomach, warms the spleen and improves eyesight

Suitable: black rice + black beans = tonifies the kidneys

Cooking Tip

As the outside of black rice has a tough seed coat, it is not easily boiled soft. If it is not well-cooked, its nutrients will not be dissolved, and eating too much can cause acute gastroenteritis. Therefore, the black rice should be soaked overnight before cooking.

Healthy Recipe
Black Rice and Red Date Porridge

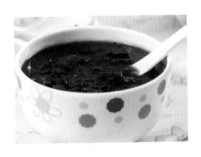

Ingredients: 80 g (3 oz) black rice, 40 g (1.5 oz) red dates, 20 g (1 oz) rice, 5 g (0.2 oz) Chinese wolfberries, 5 g (0.2 oz) white sugar, 500 g (18 oz) water

Preparation: ❶Wash the black rice clean and soak it for four hours; then rinse the rice again and soak it for 30 minutes; wash the red dates before removing their kernels; wash the Chinese wolfberries. ❷Bring a pot of water to a boil over high heat and add black rice, rice and red dates to boil them. Then cook them into a porridge on low heat. Add Chinese wolfberries and cook them for five minutes before seasoning with white sugar.

Pearl Barley

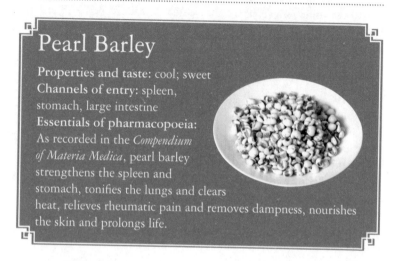

Properties and taste: cool; sweet
Channels of entry: spleen, stomach, large intestine
Essentials of pharmacopoeia:
As recorded in the *Compendium of Materia Medica*, pearl barley strengthens the spleen and stomach, tonifies the lungs and clears heat, relieves rheumatic pain and removes dampness, nourishes the skin and prolongs life.

Health Effects

Reducing blood glucose: The water extract of pearl barley effectively reduces blood glucose, and it can be processed into health-care products for reducing blood glucose.

Preventing cancer: Pearl barley contains selenium, and it effectively inhibits proliferation of cancer cells; it can be taken as adjuvant therapy for gastric cancer and cervical cancer.

Removing freckles: Pearl barley contains vitamin E, and frequent consumption makes skin smooth and supple; it also removes acne and freckles to improve skin tone.

Curing beriberi: Pearl barley is rich in vitamin B_1, and it works in preventing and curing beriberi.

Easing swelling and removing dampness: Pearl barley tonifies the spleen and clears dampness, improves kidney functions, and also clears internal heat and facilitates urination, so it has a therapeutic effect on diseases such as edema caused by nephropathy. It also produces a curative effect on diseases such as chronic enteritis and dyspepsia.

Points of Attention for Different People

Suitable for patients with tumors: Pearl barley helps relieve the adverse effects of radiotherapy and chemotherapy on patients with tumors.

Not suitable for pregnant women: It tends to cause uterine contraction, leading to abortion or premature delivery.

Food Compatibility and Incompatibility

Suitable: pearl barley + white fungus = tonifies the spleen and stomach

Suitable: pearl barley + longans = improves dry and rough skin

Suitable: pearl barley + dried bean curd = reduces cholesterol

Avoid: pearl barley + kelp = destroys vitamin E in pearl barley

Cooking Tip

It is difficult to cook pearl barley thoroughly, so it is suggested to soak it in warm water for two to three hours, as it becomes much easier to cook once it absorbs sufficient water.

Healthy Recipe
Pearl Barley and Pumpkin Soup

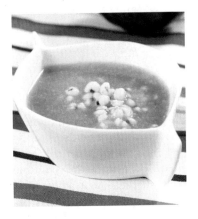

Ingredients: 100 g (3.5 oz) pearl barley, 200 g (7 oz) pumpkin, 50 g (2 oz) carrot, 200 g (7 oz) water, 10 g (0.4 oz) each white sugar and milk

Preparation: ❶Wash the pearl barley and soak in warm water until soft; peel and core the pumpkin, cut it into small cubes and wash them, steam them until they are cooked, then blend the cooked pumpkin cubes in a blender and turn them into mash. Wash the carrots and cut them into big cubes. ❷Bring carrot cubes and water to a boil, and cook for 20 minutes. Remove carrots from the pot and set them aside; put the pearl barley into the pot and bring to a boil. ❸Add the cooked pumpkin mash to the pot and season the soup with white sugar and milk.

Glutinous Rice

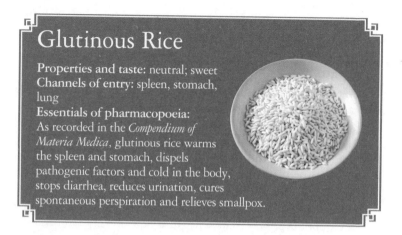

Properties and taste: neutral; sweet
Channels of entry: spleen, stomach, lung
Essentials of pharmacopoeia:
As recorded in the *Compendium of Materia Medica*, glutinous rice warms the spleen and stomach, dispels pathogenic factors and cold in the body, stops diarrhea, reduces urination, cures spontaneous perspiration and relieves smallpox.

Health Effects

Strengthening the spleen and stomach functions: Glutinous rice is gentle in its properties and taste, and it's known as "fruit of spleen." The B vitamins it contains warm the stomach and spleen, tonify qi and build up the body.

Warming the stomach and dispelling cold: Glutinous rice is a gentle tonic, and it has therapeutic effects on diseases such as gastric disorder, loss of appetite, diarrhea and frequent micturition caused by deficiency of positive qi and cold in the spleen and stomach.

Points of Attention for Different People

Suitable for patients with diarrhea: Glutinous rice warms and invigorates the spleen and stomach and has a good supplementary therapeutic effect on diarrhea.

Suitable for pregnant women: It relieves symptoms of women during the gestation period such as a strained feeling in waist and belly, shortness of breath, weakness, etc.

Not suitable for elderly people and children: Glutinous rice does not digest easily; do not eat too much at a time.

Food Compatibility and Incompatibility

Suitable: glutinous rice + red dates = relieves weakness, feebleness, palpitation and insomnia

Suitable: glutinous rice + lotus seeds = strengthens bones and teeth

Avoid: glutinous rice + eel = both are high in phosphorus, so when combined they can cause unbalanced proportions of calcium and phosphorus

Cooking Tip

To cook porridge with glutinous rice, add rice to boiling water and stir it several times before covering the pot. Bring the glutinous rice to a boil over high heat, then reduce the heat to low. Open the pot cover to stir once every ten minutes. This will give the porridge a better taste.

Healthy Recipe
Glutinous Rice and Wheat
Porridge
Ingredients: 30 g (1 oz) each glutinous rice and wheat berries, 15 g (0.5 oz) peanuts

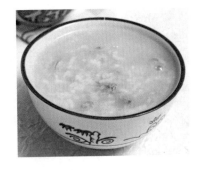

    Preparation: ❶ Wash the wheat berries and soak them for one hour; wash the glutinous rice and soak it for four hours; wash the peanuts and soak them for four hours. ❷Bring 500 g (18 oz) water to a boil in a pot. Add wheat berries and peanuts and return to a boil over high heat. Add glutinous rice to the soup and adjust to low heat to stew it for another 30 minutes, until the grains are well-cooked and soft.

Oat

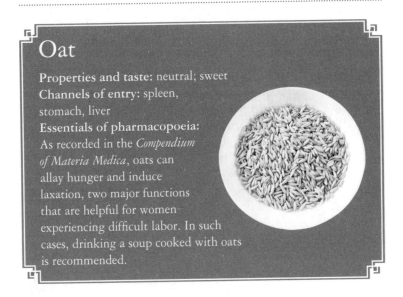

Properties and taste: neutral; sweet
Channels of entry: spleen, stomach, liver
Essentials of pharmacopoeia: As recorded in the *Compendium of Materia Medica*, oats can allay hunger and induce laxation, two major functions that are helpful for women experiencing difficult labor. In such cases, drinking a soup cooked with oats is recommended.

Health Effects

Helping to lose weight and decrease lipids: Oats are rich in soluble dietary fiber, which absorbs a large amount of cholesterol and promotes its excretion from the human body. Dietary fiber leads to satiety, so it is suggested that those obese people with abnormal blood lipid levels eat it often.

Lubricating the intestine and relaxing the bowel: The rich dietary fiber contained in oats helps gastrointestinal peristalsis, lubricates the intestines and relaxes the bowels. Many elderly people suffer from dry feces, which often causes risks to the brain's blood vessels, so eating oats is suggested for constipation relief.

Reducing blood glucose: Oats contain linoleic acid, which can effectively reduce cholesterol in the human body. Oats are rich in nutrients, and have high dietary fiber and low sugar, an ideal combination for patients with diabetes.

Points of Attention for Different People

Suitable for patients with diabetes: Oats are rich in dietary fiber, which helps control blood glucose level.

Food Compatibility and Incompatibility

Suitable: oat + yams = builds up the body and lengthens life

Suitable: oat + lily bulbs = moistens the lungs and relieves coughing

Avoid: oat + spinach = affects the absorption of calcium

Cooking Tip

The key to preparing oatmeal is to avoid boiling it for a long time over high heat, as this destroys its vitamins. The cooking time for raw oats is 20 to 30 minutes, while processed oats only require five minutes. Processed oats cooked with warm milk are done in just three minutes, and it is helpful to stir the mixture once during cooking.

Healthy Recipe

Milk and Oatmeal Drink

Ingredients: 20 g (1 oz) oatmeal, 100 g (3.5 oz) milk, one egg, 500 g (18 oz) water

Preparation: ❶Put water and oatmeal in a pot and bring

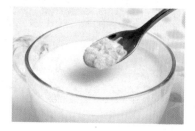

it to a boil over high heat. ❷Lower the heat to medium, beat the egg and add it to the soup. Turn off the stove and pour the soup into a bowl when the egg coagulates. ❸Add some milk (either hot or cold) to the egg and oatmeal and stir it.

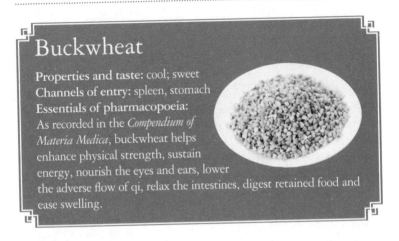

Buckwheat

Properties and taste: cool; sweet
Channels of entry: spleen, stomach
Essentials of pharmacopoeia:
As recorded in the *Compendium of Materia Medica*, buckwheat helps enhance physical strength, sustain energy, nourish the eyes and ears, lower the adverse flow of qi, relax the intestines, digest retained food and ease swelling.

Health Effects

Anti-microbial and diminishing inflammation: Buckwheat contains flavonoids that are anti-microbial and help reduce inflammation, relieve coughing and asthma, and eliminate phlegm. This grain is known as the "inflammation killer."

Reducing blood lipids and cholesterol: The magnesium, nicotinic acid and rutin found in buckwheat help reduce blood lipid and cholesterol levels.

Reducing blood glucose: The buckwheat is rich in dietary fiber and helps enhance glucose tolerance and inhibit the rise of postprandial blood sugar, so it is quite beneficial to the diabetics.

Points of Attention for Different People

Suitable for patients with diabetes: Not only does buckwheat alleviate hunger, but it also reduces blood glucose, and this therapeutic effect is quite significant.

Suitable for patients with hypertension: Buckwheat helps reduce frangibility of blood capillaries and improve micro-circulation.

Not suitable for people of allergic physique: Buckwheat

contains allergens, so it can cause or aggravate allergic symptoms.

Food Compatibility and Incompatibility
Suitable: buckwheat + yogurt = reduces cholesterol
   Suitable: buckwheat + egg = improves health of skin and nervous system
   Suitable: buckwheat + rice = provides inter-complementary nutrients
   Avoid: buckwheat + yellow croaker = affects digestion

Cooking Tip
Buckwheat has a rough taste, which can be improved if it is cooked with rice. More importantly, buckwheat contains little lysine while rice is rich in lysine, and they complement each other nutritionally if they are cooked together. Do not eat too much buckwheat at a time, though, or it can cause indigestion.

Healthy Recipe
Buckwheat Noodles
Ingredients: 100 g (3.5 oz) buckwheat noodles; 15 g (0.5 oz) each shredded seaweed, peeled and dried shrimp and spinach; 3 g (0.1 oz) chopped green onions; 200 g (7 oz) soup-stock; 500 g (18 oz) water

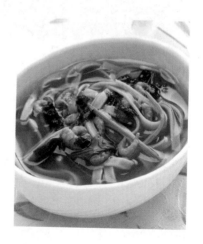

   Preparation: ❶Trim and wash the spinach, give it a quick boil and remove from the water. Cut spinach into strips; clean the peeled and dried shrimp. ❷Add the buckwheat noodles to a pot of boiling water and cook until well-done, then drain. ❸Pour soup-stock into a stockpot and bring it to a boil, add cooked buckwheat noodles to the soup, then add peeled and dried shrimp, spinach strips and shredded seaweed. Adjust the heat to the low and wait for two minutes. Get the noodles out and season them with chopped green onion.

Soybean

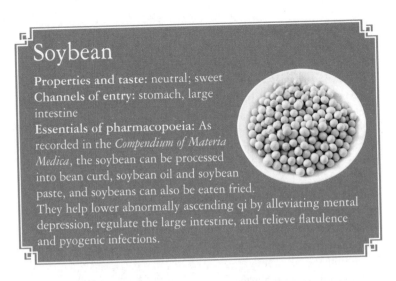

Properties and taste: neutral; sweet
Channels of entry: stomach, large intestine
Essentials of pharmacopoeia: As recorded in the *Compendium of Materia Medica*, the soybean can be processed into bean curd, soybean oil and soybean paste, and soybeans can also be eaten fried. They help lower abnormally ascending qi by alleviating mental depression, regulate the large intestine, and relieve flatulence and pyogenic infections.

Health Effects

Preventing cancer and supplementing calcium: The soybean is rich in saponin, proteinase inhibitors, isoflavones, molybdenum, selenium and other anticancer components, so it has an inhibiting effect on cancer cells. The soybean is also rich in calcium, and it has a considerable curative effect on climacteric osteoporosis.

Nourishing the brain: The soybean contains up to 40 percent protein, and the protein is a complete protein; the contained lecithin is an important element of brain cells, and it is quite effective in enhancing and improving brain function.

Expelling toxins and protecting the skin: The soybean is rich in iron, which can prevent anemia. It is quite helpful in improving rough, dry skin and dry hair, and it can also improve cell metabolism and help the body eliminate toxins. The soybean also contains more isoflavone than any other bean, so it is ideal food for women and frequent consumption is suggested.

Points of Attention for Different People

Suitable for pregnant women: Food made of soybeans can relieve the calcium loss women experience during pregnancy.

Suitable for children: The soybean is rich in iron, and can prevent and cure iron-deficiency anemia.

Not suitable for people with dyspepsia and abdominal distension: Consumption of soybeans can cause excess gas production and aggravate dyspepsia and abdominal distension.

Food Compatibility and Incompatibility

Suitable: soybeans + pine nuts = anti-aging

　Suitable: soybeans + corn = promotes digestion

　Avoid: soybeans + spinach = causes poor copper metabolism

　Avoid: soybeans + yogurt = affects the digestion and the calcium absorption rate

Cooking Tip

When cooking the soybean, make sure it's well-cooked, as undercooked soybeans may cause symptoms such as abdominal distension, diarrhea, vomiting and fever.

Healthy Recipe

Millet and Soybeans Porridge

Ingredients: 100 g (3.5 oz) millet, 50 g (2 oz) soybeans, 500 g (18 oz) water

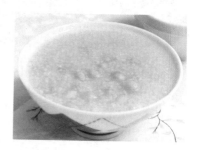

　Preparation: ❶Wash the soybeans and soak them for four hours; wash the millet. ❷Bring a pot of water to a boil, add the soybeans and cook over high heat until they are well-cooked. Adjust the heat to low and simmer until the soybeans become soft and tender; add the millet to the pot and cook it slowly over low heat; the porridge is done when it becomes sticky.

Black Bean

Properties and taste: neutral; sweet

Channels of entry: spleen, kidney

Essentials of pharmacopoeia:
As recorded in the *Compendium of Materia Medica*, the black bean can cure edema due to spleen deficiency, relieve flatulence, lower abnormally ascending qi, dispel wind-heat, and promote the blood circulation and detoxication.

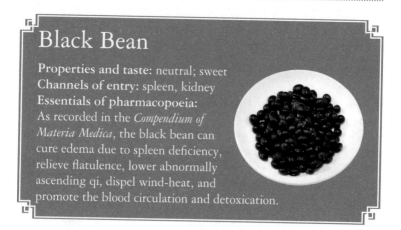

Health Effects

Tonifying and nourishing the kidney: Black bean consumption can relieve symptoms such as frequent urination, soreness of the waist, abnormal vaginal discharge, and a cold feeling in the lower belly for people with kidney deficiencies.

Protecting and nourishing the skin: Black beans are rich in vitamin E, anthocyanin and isoflavone, and their functions include clearing away the free radicals in the human body, producing anti-oxidants and skin protection; they also have a nourishing, anti-aging effect.

Invigorating the brain and promoting intelligence: The unsaturated fatty acid in black beans is transformed into the lecithin in the human body, and its functions include preventing the aging of human brain, invigorating the brain and improving intelligence. It also has an auxiliary effect of preventing senile dementia.

Points of Attention for Different People

Suitable for patients with heart disease: Frequent intake of black beans helps soften blood vessels and is beneficial to the treatment of heart disease.

Suitable for patients with diabetes: The glycemic index of the black bean is quite low.

Not suitable for people with dyspepsia: Too much intake of black beans will cause difficult digestion.

Food Compatibility and Incompatibility

Suitable: black beans + brown sugar = warms the stomach, nourish the skin, tonifies the liver and kidneys

Suitable: black beans + carp = alleviates water retention and eases swelling

Avoid: black beans + castor bean = may cause uncomfortable symptoms

Cooking Tip

Do not eat black beans unless they are well-cooked, because the black bean contains a kind of antitrypsin, which affects the digestion and absorption of protein and causes diarrhea. When the black bean is well-cooked by boiling, frying or steaming, the antitrypsin is damaged, and the side effect of the black bean is removed.

Healthy Recipe
Black Beans and Black Rice
Porridge
Ingredients: 75 g (3 oz) black
rice, 50 g (2 oz) black beans,
500 g (18 oz) water, 5 g (0.2 oz)
white sugar

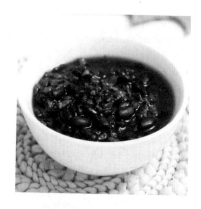

    Preparation: ❶ Wash the
black beans and black rice and
soak them each for four hours.
❷Bring a pot of water to a boil
over high heat; add the black rice
and black beans to the water and return to a full boil, then reduce the
heat to low and wait one hour until they are well-cooked; sprinkle the
porridge with white sugar and mix it evenly.

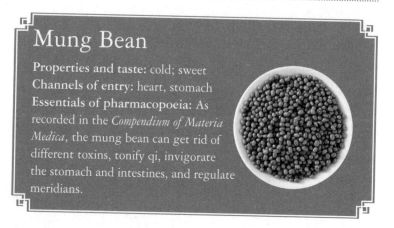

Mung Bean

Properties and taste: cold; sweet
Channels of entry: heart, stomach
Essentials of pharmacopoeia: As
recorded in the *Compendium of Materia
Medica*, the mung bean can get rid of
different toxins, tonify qi, invigorate
the stomach and intestines, and regulate
meridians.

Health Effects

Relieving summer heat and eliminating toxins: The functions
of mung bean include clearing internal heat, getting rid of toxins,
activating blood and dissolving stasis, clearing summer heat, and
curing fever, internal heat and all kinds of diseases caused by summer
heat.

    Promoting urination and detumescence: Mung beans are cold
in property and sweet in taste and can eliminate water-dampness and
cure all kinds of edema. Their functions also include antianaphylaxis,

and they can cure conditions such as hives.

Clearing away the heart fire and improving eyesight: Mung beans help clear away the heart fire, improve eyesight and produce an anti-hypertensive effect if people use a pillow stuffed with dried mung bean coatings.

Points of Attention for Different People

Suitable for patients with hypertension: Frequent intake of mung beans reduces blood pressure.

Suitable for the people with hot constitutions: The mung bean can clear summer heat, relieve restlessness, moisten dryness and disperse toxic-heat.

Not suitable for people with weak spleen and stomach: The mung bean is cool in property, and those with weak spleen and stomach should not eat too much.

Not suitable for patients under medication: The mung bean may reduce pharmaceutical effects of medication.

Food Compatibility and Incompatibility

Suitable: mung beans + lily bulbs = clears internal heat and detoxifies

Suitable: mung beans + pumpkins = relieves dizziness and weakness

Suitable: mung beans + pearl barley = improves skin tone and cures beriberi

Avoid: mung beans + alkali = destroys B vitamins

Cooking Tip

Do not cook mung beans in an iron pot. The mung bean contains tannic acid, which reacts with the iron element, and the generated iron tannate not only affects appetite and flavor but is also detrimental to the human body.

Healthy Recipe

Mung Beans and Milk Jelly

Ingredients: 30 g (1 oz) mung beans, 250 ml (8.5 oz) milk, 10 g (0.4 oz) red dates, 10 g (0.4 oz) agar, 5 g (0.2 oz) white sugar

Preparation: ❶Wash the mung beans and red dates and soak them for four hours; put them in a pressure cooker until they are cooked, and soak the agar in hot water. ❷Pour the milk into the pot and bring it to a boil; add white sugar to it until it is dissolved, then add the agar to the boiling milk. ❸Turn off the stove after three minutes of cooking over low heat; add the cooked mung beans and red dates and mix it up evenly; pour it into a glass until cooled, and it is done when it coagulates.

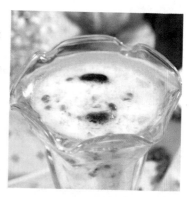

Red Bean

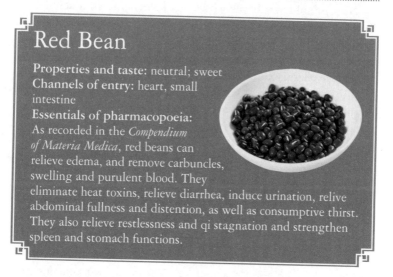

Properties and taste: neutral; sweet
Channels of entry: heart, small intestine
Essentials of pharmacopoeia:
As recorded in the *Compendium of Materia Medica*, red beans can relieve edema, and remove carbuncles, swelling and purulent blood. They eliminate heat toxins, relieve diarrhea, induce urination, relive abdominal fullness and distention, as well as consumptive thirst. They also relieve restlessness and qi stagnation and strengthen spleen and stomach functions.

Health Effects

Promoting urination and detoxifying: Red beans are rich in saponin, which stimulates the intestinal tract, promoting urination and dispelling the effects of alcohol.

Diminishing inflammation and detoxifying the body: Red beans can be used to cure traumatic injuries, blood stasis and pain, as they can diminish inflammation and detoxify the body.

Eliminating edema: Red beans are an ideal food for patients with all kinds of edema, such as cardiogenic and renal edema, ascites due to cirrhosis, and beriberi edema; they can also serve as auxiliary food therapy for people with edema type obesity.

Promoting lactation: Red beans are rich in folic acid, and their functions include eliminating dampness, promoting urination, and promoting lactation.

Points of Attention for Different People
Suitable for patients with edema and kidney inflammation: Red beans have functions such as diuresis, easing swelling and providing an anti-hypertensive effect.

Suitable for parturient and breastfeeding women: Red beans have the function of promoting lactation.

Not suitable for people with frequent urination: Red beans aggravate the symptoms of this condition.

Food Compatibility and Incompatibility
Suitable: red beans + lily bulbs = benefits qi and nourishes blood, tranquilizes nerves

Suitable: red beans + carp = induces urination and eliminates dampness

Avoid: red beans + mutton = reduces the warming and invigorating efficacy of mutton

Cooking Tip
The red bean contains an enzyme known as "flatulence factor," which causes aerogenesis of the intestinal tract, leading to flatulence. Adding some salt when the red beans are cooking helps diminish this flatulence.

Healthy Recipe
Red Beans and Pearl Barley Paste
Ingredients: 50 g (2 oz) pearl barley, 20 g (1 oz) rice, 20 g (1 oz) red beans, 10 g (0.4 oz) rock sugar

Preparation: ❶Wash rice, pearl barley and red beans, and soak them for five to six hours. ❷Pour rice, pearl barley and red beans into the automatic soy milk maker and add water reaches 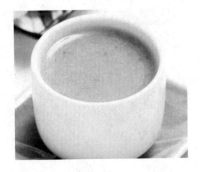 between the upper and lower water lines. Wait until the soybean milk machine indicates that the paste is done; stir the rock sugar into the paste until the sugar is dissolved.

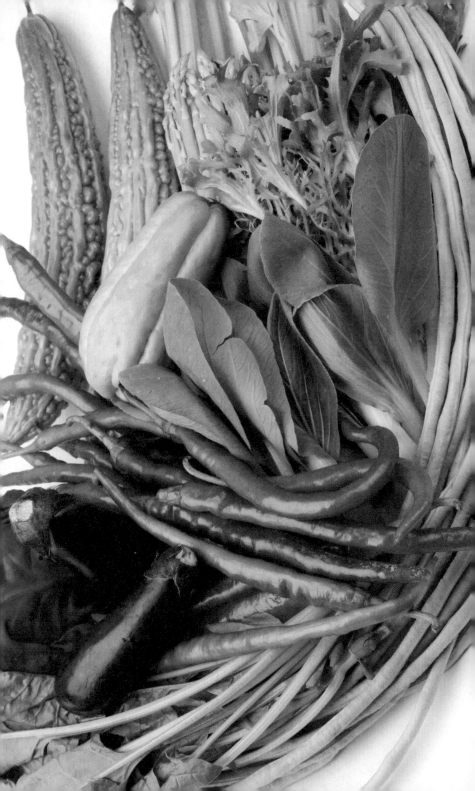

Chapter Three
Vegetables

Vegetables are not only rich in vitamins, dietary fiber, calcium, phosphorus, iron and trace elements like zinc, selenium, and iodine, they also contain many phytochemicals that are very beneficial to the human body (such as soy isoflavones in soybeans, garlic extract in garlic, etc.). They can fight oxidation and improve other vitamins' physiological functions. Vegetables provide necessary nutrients for the human body while also offering good disease prevention and curative effects.

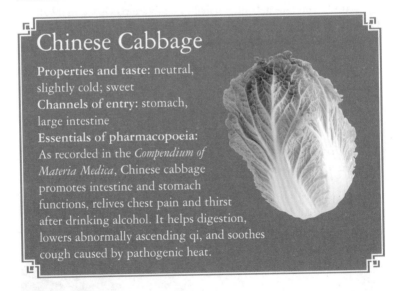

Chinese Cabbage

Properties and taste: neutral, slightly cold; sweet
Channels of entry: stomach, large intestine
Essentials of pharmacopoeia:
As recorded in the *Compendium of Materia Medica*, Chinese cabbage promotes intestine and stomach functions, relives chest pain and thirst after drinking alcohol. It helps digestion, lowers abnormally ascending qi, and soothes cough caused by pathogenic heat.

Health Effects
Lubricating the intestine and relaxing the bowel: Chinese cabbage is rich in dietary fiber, and it not only lubricates the intestines, relaxes the bowels and promotes the expulsion of toxins, but also stimulates gastrointestinal peristalsis and digestion, which helps prevent intestinal cancer.

Preventing cardiovascular disease: Chinese cabbage is rich in vitamin C, and it clears heat, dispels fire, nourishes the stomach and promotes the secretion of body fluids. It also reduces cholesterol levels, improves vascular elasticity, and helps prevent cardiovascular disease.

Points of Attention for Different People
Suitable for people with abdominal distension: Chinese cabbage promotes the functions of the intestines and stomach, which is ideal for people with abdominal distension.

Food Compatibility and Incompatibility
Suitable: Chinese cabbage + tomatoes = prevents against cold and relieves pressure

Suitable: Chinese cabbage + cheese = prevents osteoporosis

Suitable: Chinese cabbage + lean meat = brightens the skin and eliminates fatigue

Avoid: Chinese cabbage + cucumbers = damages vitamin C in Chinese cabbage

Avoid: Chinese cabbage + pork liver = affects the absorption of vitamin C

Cooking Tip
It's best not to soak Chinese cabbage for a long time, as its water-soluble vitamins can dissolve in water and its original nutritive value lost. Also, avoid cooking Chinese cabbage with cookware made of copper, in case the vitamin C it contains is damaged by cupric ion and its nutritive value is reduced.

Healthy Recipe
Sweet and Sour Chinese Cabbage

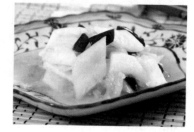

Ingredients: 500 g (18 oz) outer leaves of cabbage; 3 g (0.1 oz) each salt, white sugar, vinegar, water starch, chopped scallion, Sichuan peppers, and dried chilis; 10 g (0.4 oz) vegetable oil

Preparation: ❶Wash the outer leaves of the cabbage and cut them into rhombus shapes; pickle the cabbage with salt and squeeze off the moisture. ❷Prepare a sauce by mixing salt, white sugar, vinegar, chopped scallions and water starch in a small bowl. ❸Heat the oil in a wok and add the Sichuan peppers to the pan, stir-fry and remove for later use. Put the dried chilis in the pan and fry until the color turns maroon, then add the Chinese cabbage to the wok and fry it over high heat until it is cooked. Add the sauce, and the dish is done when the soup becomes thick.

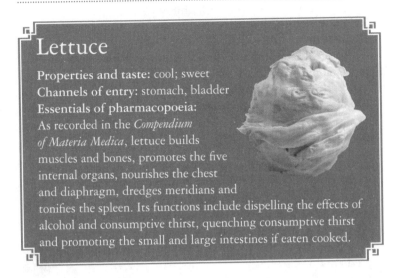

Lettuce

Properties and taste: cool; sweet
Channels of entry: stomach, bladder
Essentials of pharmacopoeia:
As recorded in the *Compendium of Materia Medica*, lettuce builds muscles and bones, promotes the five internal organs, nourishes the chest and diaphragm, dredges meridians and tonifies the spleen. Its functions include dispelling the effects of alcohol and consumptive thirst, quenching consumptive thirst and promoting the small and large intestines if eaten cooked.

Health Effects
Losing weight: Lettuce is rich in moisture, dietary fiber and vitamin C, and it helps remove excessive fat from the human body, so it is known as an "anti-obesity food."

Improving sleep quality: The stem leaf of lettuce contains lactucin, whose functions include clearing heat, diminishing inflammation, analgesia, hypnosis, reducing cholesterol, serving as adjuvant therapy of neurasthenia and so on.

Promoting urination: Effective components such as mannitol are found in the stem leaf of lettuce; these have functions such as diuresis and stimulating blood circulation.

Points of Attention for Different People
Suitable for obese people: Lettuce is rich in dietary fiber, and it helps eliminate excess fat.

Suitable for patients with hyperlipemia: The stem leaf contains lactucin, so it helps reduce cholesterol.

Suitable for people with difficult urination: The lettuce contains mannitol, with the effects of stimulating both diuresis and blood circulation.

Not suitable for people with weakness of the spleen and the stomach functions: Lettuce is cold in properties.

Food Compatibility and Incompatibility

Suitable: lettuce + rabbit meat = promotes the absorption rate and digestion of nutrients

Suitable: lettuce + garlic = clears heat, removes toxicity, and improves immunity

Suitable: lettuce + bean curd = expels toxins and nourishes the skin

Avoid: lettuce + vinegar = reduces nutritive value

Cooking Tip

Do not cut lettuce with a metal kitchen knife because when the two are in contact, the cuts on the lettuce will turn brown and the taste is reduced. For a better flavor, break the leaves off by hand one by one and tear them into pieces of the proper size.

Healthy Recipes

Lettuce and Watermelon Juice

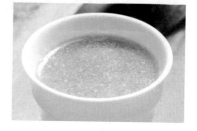

Ingredients: 100 g (3.5 oz) lettuce, 50 g (2 oz) watermelon flesh, 5 g (0.2 oz) honey, 100 g (3.5 oz) drinking water

Preparation: ❶Wash the lettuce and tear it into small pieces; core and dice the watermelon. ❷Put the lettuce and watermelon into a juicer, add some drinking water to the machine for blending, and stir some honey into the juice.

Soy Milk with Kiwi and Lettuce

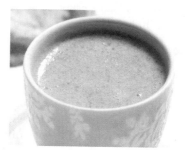

Ingredients: 150 g (5 oz) kiwi, 100 g (3.5 oz) lettuce, 300 ml (10 oz) soy milk

Preparation: ❶Peel and dice the kiwi; wash the lettuce and tear it into pieces. ❷Put the above ingredients and the soy milk into a juicer.

Cabbage

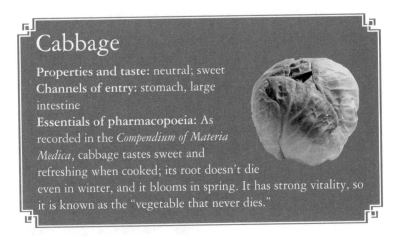

Properties and taste: neutral; sweet
Channels of entry: stomach, large intestine
Essentials of pharmacopoeia: As recorded in the *Compendium of Materia Medica*, cabbage tastes sweet and refreshing when cooked; its root doesn't die even in winter, and it blooms in spring. It has strong vitality, so it is known as the "vegetable that never dies."

Health Effects

Preventing cancer: Nitrosamines are typical carcinogens. Cabbage contains an enzyme that decomposes nitrosamines, which can suppress the mutagenesis of nitrosamines. Besides, the microelements in cabbage help inhibit synthesis of nitrosamines.

Anti-bacteria and diminishing inflammation: Fresh cabbage helps relieve uncomfortable symptoms such as throat pain, pain caused by injuries, mosquito bites, stomachache and toothache.

Expelling toxins and losing weight: Cabbage has an even higher iodine content than most seafood, so it is helpful in expelling toxins and facilitating weight loss.

Points of Attention for Different People

Not suitable for people with diarrhea: Cabbage is rich in fiber, but the fiber is quite rough and does not digest easily.

Food Compatibility and Incompatibility

Suitable: cabbage + pork = makes skin feel soft and supple

Suitable: cabbage + bamboo shoots = stimulates blood circulation

Suitable: cabbage + mayonnaise = improves skin, has anti-aging and anti-cancer properties

Avoid: cabbage + cucumbers = destroys vitamin C

Avoid: cabbage + honey = reduces nutritive value

Cooking Tip

Cabbage contains water-soluble vitamins, so to avoid loss of nutrients, it's best not to cut it too finely before washing or soaking. To make sure that the nutrients in cabbage are better absorbed, it can be made into all kinds of salads or cold dishes. Cook the cabbage in boiling water for just a short time to avoid nutrient loss.

Healthy Recipe

Stewed Cabbage with Beef Slices

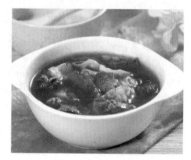

Ingredients: 250 g (9 oz) beef; 150 g (5 oz) tomatoes; 150 g (5 oz) cabbage; 3 g (0.1 oz) each rice wine, salt, monosodium glutamate and vegetable oil

Preparation: ❶Wash and dice the tomatoes; trim and wash the cabbage and cut it into slices; wash the beef and cut it into thin slices. ❷Put the beef slices into the pot with some water, and bring to a boil over high heat; remove floating foam, and add vegetable oil and rice wine. Boil until the beef is almost done; put tomatoes and cabbage into the pan and stew them until they are cooked; season them with salt and monosodium glutamate and continue to stew for a few more minutes.

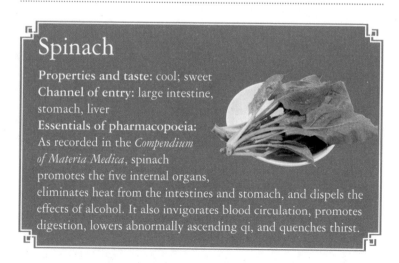

Spinach

Properties and taste: cool; sweet
Channel of entry: large intestine, stomach, liver
Essentials of pharmacopoeia:
As recorded in the *Compendium of Materia Medica*, spinach promotes the five internal organs, eliminates heat from the intestines and stomach, and dispels the effects of alcohol. It also invigorates blood circulation, promotes digestion, lowers abnormally ascending qi, and quenches thirst.

Health Effects

Reducing blood glucose: Spinach leaves contain a substance like insulin, which can help patients with type II diabetes to maintain balanced blood sugar levels.

Lubricating the intestine and relaxing the bowel: Spinach is rich in dietary fiber, which helps promote intestinal tract movement and defecation, and has a good curative effect on hemorrhoids and constipation.

Points of Attention for Different People

Suitable for patients with diabetes: The spinach leaves contain a substance similar to insulin and helps maintain balanced blood sugar levels.

Suitable for people with constipation: Spinach helps clear away heat toxins of the intestines and stomach and prevent constipation.

Not suitable for people with diarrhea: Spinach is cool in properties, and it tends to cause laxation.

Food Compatibility and Incompatibility

Suitable: spinach + garlic = eliminates fatigue

Suitable: spinach + kelp = good for bones and teeth

Suitable: spinach + eggs = helps maintain the balance between calcium and phosphorus

Avoid: spinach + walnuts = leads to lithiasis

Avoid: spinach + cheese = affects the absorption rate of calcium

Cooking Tip

Spinach is rich in oxalic acid, and excessive consumption will prevent the human body from utilizing iron and calcium, and it can even form lithiasis of the urethral canal or aggravate the symptoms of lithiasis. Therefore, before cooking, cook the spinach in boiling water briefly, then drain the spinach to prevent excessive consumption of oxalic acid.

Healthy Recipe
Peanuts and Spinach

Ingredients: 50 g (2 oz) cooked peanuts; 300 g (11 oz) spinach; 3 g (0.1 oz) each minced garlic, salt, monosodium glutamate and sesame oil; 200 g (7 oz) water

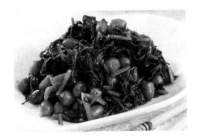

Preparation: ❶Trim and wash the spinach and add it to boiling water for 30 minutes; remove it from water and cool; drain well and cut it into strips. ❷Prepare a dish and put spinach strips and cooked peanuts into it, and season them with minced garlic, salt, monosodium glutamate and sesame oil.

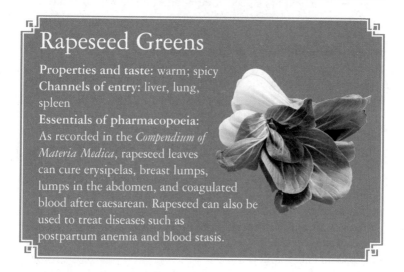

Rapeseed Greens

Properties and taste: warm; spicy
Channels of entry: liver, lung, spleen
Essentials of pharmacopoeia:
As recorded in the *Compendium of Materia Medica*, rapeseed leaves can cure erysipelas, breast lumps, lumps in the abdomen, and coagulated blood after caesarean. Rapeseed can also be used to treat diseases such as postpartum anemia and blood stasis.

Health Effects

Preventing constipation: Rapeseed greens contain dietary fiber that promotes intestinal tract movement, shortens the time feces stays in the intestinal tract, helps relax the bowels and provides adjuvant therapy for different kinds of constipation, as well as preventing tumors of the intestinal tract.

Expelling toxins and preventing cancer: Because phytohormones contained in rapeseed leaves facilitate the formation of enzymes, absorb and decompose the cancerogenic substances that enter human body, rapeseed greens' functions include cancer prevention. The rapeseed greens also enhances the liver's detoxification mechanism, so its functions include detoxification and easing swelling.

Points of Attention for Different People

Suitable for beauty pursuers: It helps resist hyperkeratosis.

Suitable for parturients: It provides adjuvant therapy for postpartum blood stasis and stomachache.

Suitable for patients with pancreatic cancer: Rapeseed greens help reduce the morbidity of pancreatic cancer.

Food Compatibility and Incompatibility

Suitable: rapeseed greens + mushrooms = helps prevent cancer

Suitable: rapeseed greens + shrimp = improves calcium absorption, tonifies kidneys and yang

Suitable: rapeseed greens + bean curd = relieves cough and asthma and enhances immunity

Avoid: rapeseed greens + yams = affects the absorption of nutrients

Avoid: rapeseed greens + pumpkins = reduces the nutritive value of rapeseed leaves

Cooking Tip

It is recommended to cook rapeseed greens in cooking oil, as the oil enables the rapeseed's fat-soluble nutrients to be better absorbed by the human body. If boiling the greens, achieve the same effect by adding some sesame oil to the soup.

Healthy Recipes

Sesame and Rapeseed Leaves

Ingredients: 150 g (5 oz) rapeseed greens; 25 g (1 oz) white sesame; 3 g (0.1 oz) each salt, sesame oil and monosodium glutamate

Preparation: ❶Trim and wash the rapeseed leaves and scald them in boiling water for one minute; remove, cool, and drain well; remove impurities from the white sesame. ❷Heat the white sesame in a pan, stir-fry until cooked, remove from the pan and let it cool. ❸Prepare a dish and put the rapeseed into it; add salt, monosodium glutamate and sesame oil and mix evenly; serve garnished with a sprinkle of cooked white sesame.

Mushrooms and Rapeseed Leaves

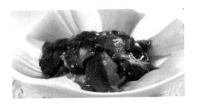

Ingredients: 200 g (7 oz) rapeseed greens; 100 g (3.5 oz) mushrooms; 20 g (1 oz) each chopped green onion, Sichuan pepper powder, cornstarch, salt, monosodium glutamate and vegetable oil.

Preparation: ❶Trim and wash the rapeseed leaves; remove the roots of fresh mushrooms and tear them into small pieces. Put mushrooms into boiling water; and remove when softened. ❷Heat vegetable oil in a wok, then add chopped green onions and Sichuan pepper powder and stir-fry until fragrant and the oil is 70 percent heated, when a large amount of smoke is rising from the oil. ❸Put the rapeseed and fresh mushrooms into the pan and stir-fry them for four minutes; thicken with a mixture of cornstarch and water; complete the dish by seasoning it with monosodium glutamate and salt.

Food Note

Rapeseed is used in some countries mainly in the form of canola oil. The greens are a common ingredient in TCM cooking but can be hard to find. Their Latin name is Brassica napus L., and seeds are readily available. Try a local Asian market for these greens.

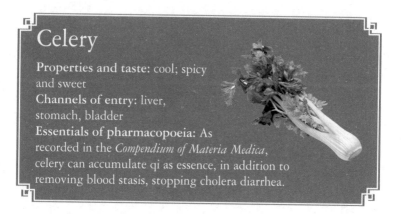

Celery

Properties and taste: cool; spicy and sweet
Channels of entry: liver, stomach, bladder
Essentials of pharmacopoeia: As recorded in the *Compendium of Materia Medica*, celery can accumulate qi as essence, in addition to removing blood stasis, stopping cholera diarrhea.

Health Effects
Lowering blood pressure and clearing the bowel: Celery petioles are plump and tender, rich in minerals, vitamins and mannitol, which can not only increase appetite, but also have the effects of lowering blood pressure, clearing the bowels and facilitating urination.

Maintaining beauty and anti-cancer: Celery contains a large amount of dietary fiber, which can stimulate gastrointestinal motility, promote bowel movements and clear the bowels. It is a good product for weight-reduction and beauty. It can also reduce the contact between carcinogens and colonic mucosa to prevent colon cancer.

Points of Attention for Different People

Suitable for people with constipation: Celery contains a large amount of crude fiber, which can stimulate gastrointestinal motility and promote bowel movements.

Suitable for hypertensive patients: Celery protects blood vessels and has an auxiliary therapeutic effect on hypertension and vascular sclerosis.

Not suitable for people with low blood pressure: As celery has the effect of lowering blood pressure, those with low blood pressure should be careful when eating it.

Food Compatibility and Incompatibility

Suitable: celery + octopus = strengthens the heart, protects the liver, and reduces cholesterol

Suitable: celery + olive oil = protects the eyes, has anti-cancer properties

Avoid: celery + clams = destroys vitamin B_1 in celery

Avoid: celery + honey = tends to cause diarrhea

Cooking Tip

When eating celery, most people eat the stems and petioles. In fact, its leaves have richer vitamin and mineral content than its stems and petioles, so are the most healthful part of the plant.

Healthy Recipe

Peanuts with Celery

Ingredients: 50 g (2 oz) peanuts; 200 g (7 oz) celery; 3 g (0.1 oz) each salt, monosodium glutamate and sesame oil

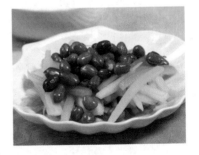

Preparation: ❶Remove impurities from peanuts, wash and cook them. Remove peanuts from the pot and set aside to drain and cool. Wash celery clean and place it into the boiling water pot to blanch. Remove celery to drain and cool it, then cut it into segments. ❷Peanuts and celery are served in a dish, and seasoned with salt, monosodium glutamate and sesame oil.

Chinese Leek

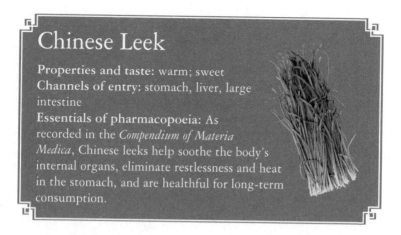

Properties and taste: warm; sweet
Channels of entry: stomach, liver, large intestine
Essentials of pharmacopoeia: As recorded in the *Compendium of Materia Medica*, Chinese leeks help soothe the body's internal organs, eliminate restlessness and heat in the stomach, and are healthful for long-term consumption.

Health Effects

Tonifying the kidney and warming yang: Leeks warm the spleen and stomach, stimulate the appetite, promote the circulation of qi and invigorate blood circulation. Their functions include tonifying the kidney, warming yang and regulating internal organs. Leek seeds can control nocturnal emissions, support yang, tonify the kidney, and warm the waist and knees, so are useful for treating diseases such as erectile dysfunction, spermatorrhea and premature ejaculation.

Lubricating the intestine and relaxing the bowel: The leek is rich in vitamin and dietary fiber, which promote gastrointestinal peristalsis and cure constipation.

Reducing blood pressure: Frequent intake of leek juice provides good adjuvant therapy for diseases such as hypertension, coronary heart disease and hyperlipemia.

Points of Attention for Different People

Suitable for people with constipation: Leeks are rich in dietary fiber, which promotes intestinal tract movement and helps defecation.

Suitable for people with cold constitution: The leek is warm in nature, and its functions include strengthening the stomach, warming the spleen, stomach and kidneys, supporting yang, dispersing blood stasis and invigorating blood circulation.

Not suitable for people with fire excess from yin deficiency: Leeks do not digest easily and can cause excessive internal heat.

Food Compatibility and Incompatibility

Suitable: leeks + sunflower seed oil = prevents cancer and heart disease

Suitable: leeks + lean meat = eliminates fatigue, enhances and brightens complexion

Avoid: leeks + honey = causes diarrhea

Avoid: leeks + vinegar = reduces nutritive value

Cooking Tip

The best leeks are grown in the early spring, followed by those grown in the late autumn, and leeks grown in summer are of the poorest quality. Therefore, there is a saying: "The leek smells fragrant in spring while it smells odorous in summer."

Healthy Recipe

Dried Shrimp with Leeks

Ingredients: 200 g (7 oz) leeks; 50 g (2 oz) shrimp meat; 20 g (1 oz) vegetable oil; 3 g (0.1 oz) each green onion, ginger and salt

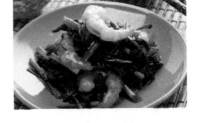

Preparation: ❶Wash the leeks and cut into strips 3 cm in length; wash the shrimp meat; cut the ginger into shreds and green onion into strips. ❷Heat some vegetable oil in a pan and wait until the oil is about 60 percent heated and a small amount of smoke comes from the pot; put shredded ginger and green onions into the pan, stir-fry until fragrant; put shrimp meat, leek and salt into the pan and stir-fry until cooked.

Tomato

Properties and taste: slightly cold; sweet

Channels of entry: lung, stomach

Essentials of pharmacopoeia: As recorded in the *Compendium of Materia Medica*, tomatoes are sweet, sour and slightly cold. They promote the secretion of saliva and body fluids, strengthen the stomach and help digestion, and they can be used to treat thirst and anorexia.

Health Effects

Lubricating the intestine and nourishing the stomach: The tomato contains organic acids such as malic acid and citric acid, and it improves the concentration of gastric acid, regulates intestine and stomach functions; the dietary fiber in tomatoes can be used to prevent and treat constipation.

Reducing blood fat and lowering blood pressure: Tomatoes contain vitamin C, rutin, lycopene and tartaric acid, which reduce blood cholesterol and prevent atherosclerosis and coronary heart disease; the potassium in tomatoes helps lowering blood pressure, promote urination and ease swelling.

Maintaining beauty and protecting the skin: Frequent tomato consumption diminishes freckles, provides an anti-aging effect and protects skin.

Points of Attention for Different People

Suitable for people with kidney deficiency: Frequent intake of tomatoes is suggested.

Suitable for beauty pursuers: Eating cooked tomatoes has good cosmetic results.

Not suitable for patients with leucoderma: Tomatoes are rich in vitamin C, which prevents the oxidization of dopamine enzyme into hallachrome, while the hallachrome helps prevent the regeneration of melanin at lesions.

Food Compatibility and Incompatibility

Suitable: tomatoes + bean curd = maintains beauty and improves immunity

Suitable: tomatoes + potatoes = stimulates blood circulation

Suitable: tomatoes + pork liver = promotes effect of iron supplements

Avoid: tomatoes + carrots = destroys vitamin C

Cooking Tip

Adding some vinegar during cooking destroys tomatidine, which is a hazardous substance contained in tomatoes. It is suggested that the tomato be stir-fried with strong heat, because its vitamins will be easily destroyed and the nutritive value will be reduced if tomatoes are subject to prolonged cooking.

Healthy Recipe
Tomato, Chinese Wolfberries and
Corn Soup
Ingredients: 200 g (7 oz) corn
kernels, 50 g (2 oz) tomatoes, 10 g
(0.4 oz) Chinese wolfberries, one
egg white, 4 g (0.2 oz) salt, 2 g
(0.1 oz) monosodium glutamate,
2 g (0.1 oz) each sesame oil and
water starch, 20 g (1 oz) tomato
soup-stock

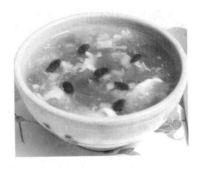

Preparation: ❶Wash the corn kernels; remove tomato stems,
then wash and dice tomatoes; wash Chinese wolfberries; whip an
egg white. ❷Heat tomato soup-stock in a pot over high heat, add
corn kernels to the soup, and bring to a boil. Adjust the heat to
medium or low and boil for five minutes. ❸Add diced tomatoes and
Chinese wolfberries to the soup and return to a boil. Thicken the soup
with water starch, add the egg white to the soup and stir; finish by
seasoning with salt and monosodium glutamate and sprinkling with
some sesame oil.

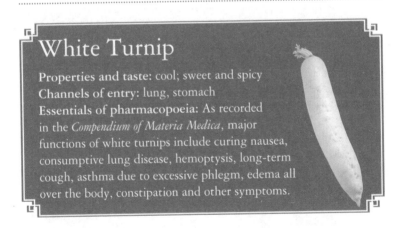

White Turnip

Properties and taste: cool; sweet and spicy
Channels of entry: lung, stomach
Essentials of pharmacopoeia: As recorded
in the *Compendium of Materia Medica*, major
functions of white turnips include curing nausea,
consumptive lung disease, hemoptysis, long-term
cough, asthma due to excessive phlegm, edema all
over the body, constipation and other symptoms.

Health Effects
Lowering blood sugar and preventing constipation: With rich
mustard oil and soluble dietary fiber, white turnips can delay food
absorption, and lower postprandial blood sugar. They can also promote
intestinal peristalsis to prevent constipation.

Invigorating the stomach and helping digestion: White turnips have a special spicy taste, which can increase appetite and help digestion.

Reducing blood fat and stabilizing blood pressure: Frequent consumption of white turnips, which are rich in potassium, can reduce blood fat, soften blood vessels and stabilize blood pressure.

Points of Attention for Different People

Suitable for immunocompromised people: Rich in vitamin C and the trace element zinc, white turnips help to enhance the body's immune function.

Suitable for people with indigestion: The mustard oil component of white turnips can promote gastrointestinal motility, increase appetite and help digestion.

Not suitable for people with weak spleen and stomach: Because white turnips are cold in properties and can lead to more bowel movements, people with diarrhea due to spleen deficiency should be careful not to eat too much white turnip.

Food Compatibility and Incompatibility

Suitable: white turnips + cabbage = maintains healthy skin

Suitable: white turnips + soybean oil = helps the body absorb calcium

Suitable: white turnips + clams = strengthens the heart and protects the liver

Avoid: white turnips + carrots = destroys vitamin C

Avoid: white turnips + honey = tends to cause diarrhea

Cooking Tip

White turnips can be eaten raw or stewed or cooked. It is better to choose juicy and less spicy white turnips when eating them raw. Those who do not like to eat cold food usually prefer cooked turnip.

Healthy Recipes

Turnip-Rib Pot

Ingredients: 250 g (9 oz) white turnip; 300 g (11 oz) pork ribs; 2 g (0.1 oz) each chopped coriander, pepper, chopped green onion, cooking wine, salt and dark soy sauce

Preparation: ❶ Wash the ribs and chop them into pieces; wash the white turnip and cut it into pieces; put both pork and turnips in boiling water and blanch them, then drain. **❷** Put the ribs and turnip pieces into a pot with some water. Bring to a boil over high heat, then reduce the heat to

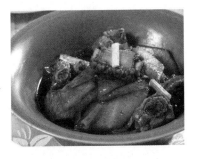

low and stew for 45 minutes. Season with salt, cooking wine, pepper and dark soy sauce, then sprinkle with chopped green onions and coriander.

White Turnip and Dark Plum Soup

Ingredients: 250 g (9 oz) fresh white turnips, two dark plums, 2 g (0.1 oz) salt, 300 g (11 oz) water

Preparation: ❶ Wash fresh white turnips and slice thinly. **❷** Put the turnips and plums into a pot and add water to cook for one to two hours over low heat. Season with salt to serve.

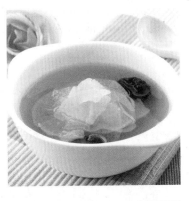

Carrot

Properties and taste: warm; sweet
Channels of entry: liver, lung, spleen
Essentials of pharmacopoeia: As recorded in the *Compendium of Materia Medica*, carrots lower abnormally ascending qi, invigorate spleen-stomach, promote the chest and diaphragm, harmonize the intestines and stomach, calm the five internal organs, promote appetite and are quite good for the human body.

Health Effects

Benefitting the liver and improving the eyesight: The carrot is rich in carotene; the human body transforms about half of it into vitamin A, which nourishes the liver and improves eyesight, and can treat nyctalopia.

Reducing blood glucose and lipid: Carrots contain substances that lower blood glucose; the quercetin and kaempferol in carrots help increase coronary blood flow and lower blood lipids. Additionally, carrots provide good dietary therapy for people with diabetes, hypertension and coronary heart disease.

Points of Attention for Different People

Suitable for patients with diabetes: Carrots contain substances that lower blood glucose.

Suitable for smokers: Carrots contain natural carotene, which helps maintain the integrity of respiratory tract mucosal tissues and protects the trachea, bronchia and lungs.

Suitable for patients with hypertension: The potassium succinate in carrots helps reduce blood pressure.

Not suitable for women of childbearing age: Excessive carotene intake may cause amenorrhea and inhibit normal ovulation.

Food Compatibility and Incompatibility

Suitable: carrots + sesame oil = protects eyesight and prevents from getting cold

Suitable: carrots + albacore = prevents arteriosclerosis

Suitable: carrots + dried mushrooms = protects eyesight and provides anti-aging function

Avoid: carrots + vinegar = destroys carotinoid

Cooking Tip

The carrot's main nutrient is beta-carotene, and it can only be absorbed by the human body when it is dissolved in grease. Ninety percent of a carrot's beta-carotene is wasted when it's eaten uncooked or steamed. To improve beta-carotene intake, it is suggested that the carrot is cut into shreds and fried with oil.

Healthy Recipes

Fried Fungus with Carrots

Ingredients: 250 g (9 oz) carrots; 50 g (2 oz) water-swollen black fungus; 2 g (0.1 oz) each chopped green onions, salt and monosodium glutamate; 30 g (1 oz) vegetable oil; 20 g (1 oz) water

Preparation: ❶Wash and shred the carrots; trim and wash the water-swollen black fungus and tear it into small pieces. ❷Heat a pan with vegetable oil; when the oil is 70 percent heated, put chopped green onion into the pan and stir-fry it until fragrant; add the carrot shreds and stir evenly. ❸Put the black fungus into the pan and add water; boil the carrot shreds until cooked, and season with salt and monosodium glutamate.

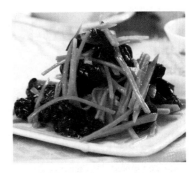

Carrots and Red Dates Soup
Ingredients: 120 g (4 oz) carrots, 40 g (1 oz) red dates, 3 g (0.1 oz) crystal sugar, 300 g (11 oz) water
Preparation: ❶Wash and slice the carrots; wash the red dates and soak them in warm water. ❷ Put carrot slices, red dates and water into the pot; boil over low heat, then season them with sugar.

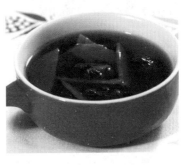

Eggplant

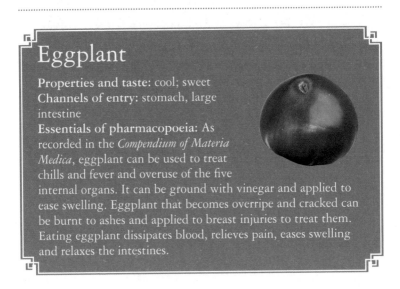

Properties and taste: cool; sweet
Channels of entry: stomach, large intestine
Essentials of pharmacopoeia: As recorded in the *Compendium of Materia Medica*, eggplant can be used to treat chills and fever and overuse of the five internal organs. It can be ground with vinegar and applied to ease swelling. Eggplant that becomes overripe and cracked can be burnt to ashes and applied to breast injuries to treat them. Eating eggplant dissipates blood, relieves pain, eases swelling and relaxes the intestines.

Health Effects

Protecting blood vessel: The eggplant is rich in flavonoids, which soften the blood vessels, enhance vascular elasticity, reduce frangibility and permeability of blood capillaries, and have a certain curative effect on diseases such as hypertension and arteriosclerosis.

Preventing and curing gastric cancer: The eggplant contains solanine, which inhibits proliferation of digestive system neoplasm, so it prevents and cures gastric cancer.

Anti-aging: The eggplant contains vitamin E, and its functions include preventing hemorrhages and providing an anti-aging effect; it also stabilizes blood cholesterol levels.

Points of Attention for Different People

Suitable for patients with hemorrhagic disease: The purple eggplant is rich in flavonoids, which improve frangibility of blood capillaries and prevent hemorrhages of small vessels.

Suitable for patients with hypercholesteremia: The saponin in eggplant reduces cholesterol.

Suitable for people with internal hemorrhoids and hemafecia: The eggplant's functions include clearing heat, invigorating blood circulation, easing swelling and relieving pain.

Not suitable for people with diarrhea: The eggplant is cool in properties, and it aggravates the symptoms of diarrhea.

Food Compatibility and Incompatibility

Suitable: eggplant + chili = brightens the skin

Suitable: eggplant + cheese = enhances the body's calcium absorption

Avoid: eggplant + hyacinth beans = affects the body's calcium absorption

Avoid: eggplant + carrots = reduces nutritive value

Cooking and Eating Tips

Try not to deep-fry the eggplant, as this cooking method can cause massive loss of flavonoids. It is not suggested to peel the eggplant, as the peel contains flavonoids and many other nutrients, and the flavonoids are concentrated in the connection between the purple peel of eggplant and its flesh.

Healthy Recipes
Steamed Eggplant

Ingredients: 500 g (18 oz) eggplant; 50 g (2 oz) water-swollen mushrooms; 2 g (0.1 oz) each monosodium glutamate, rice wine, salt, sesame oil, green onion strips and ginger slices; 30 g (1 oz) vegetable oil; 30 g (1 oz) water

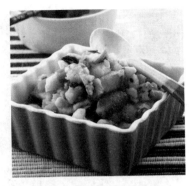

Preparation: ❶Wash, peel and dice the eggplant; wash the mushrooms and remove their stems. ❷Prepare a big bowl and load it with mushrooms and diced eggplants, sprinkling evenly with salt and monosodium glutamate. ❸Heat some oil in a pot and pour hot oil, rice wine and water into the bowl loaded with mushrooms and diced eggplant, and then add the green onion strips and ginger slices. ❹Cover the bowl, put it on a steaming tray and steam with high heat for 30 minutes; remove green onion and ginger, and sprinkle the dish with sesame oil to serve.

Fried Eggplant with Fried Tomatoes

Ingredients: 250 g (9 oz) eggplant; 50 g (2 oz) tomatoes; 2 g (0.1 oz) each chopped green onion, salt, monosodium glutamate, and water starch; 30 g (1 oz) vegetable oil; 30 g (1 oz) water

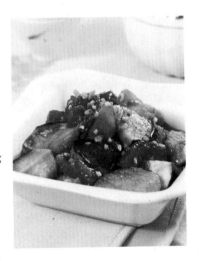

Preparation: ❶After removing the stems, wash and dice the eggplant and tomatoes. ❷Heat some vegetable oil in a pan; when the oil is 70 percent heated, add chopped green onions to the pan and stir-fry until fragrant, then add the diced eggplant and stir-fry. ❸Pour some water into the pan and boil until the diced eggplant is 80 percent cooked and chewable; add the diced tomatoes and wait until they are cooked; season with salt and monosodium glutamate and thicken with the mixture of water starch.

Green Pepper

Properties and taste: hot; spicy
Channels of entry: heart, spleen
Essentials of pharmacopoeia:
As recorded in the *Compendium of Materia Medica*, the green pepper cures food retention, regulates qi and dispels sadness, stimulates the appetite and exorcises evil spirits.

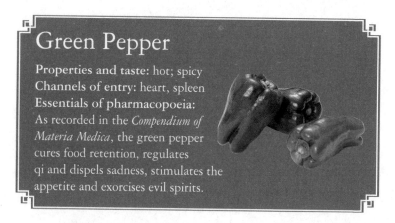

Health Effects

Stimulating the appetite and helping indigestion: The green pepper is characterized by a delicate flavor, and the capsaicin it contains stimulates secretion of saliva and gastric juices, which piques the appetite, promotes intestinal tract movement and helps indigestion.

Preventing cancer: The effective component of green pepper is capsaicin, which is an antioxidant substance that terminates the cancerous process of cells and reduces cancer morbidity.

Points of Attention for Different People

Suitable for people with anorexia: The pepper stimulates the appetite and helps indigestion.

Suitable for obese people: The capsaicin in green pepper helps promote fat metabolism, so it helps people to lose weight.

Not suitable for people with excessive internal heat: It is not suggested that patients with eye disease, esophagitis, gastroenteritis, stomach ulcers or hemorrhoids eat too much green pepper.

Food Compatibility and Incompatibility

Suitable: green peppers + chicken = hair care and skin care

Suitable: green peppers + beef = eliminates fatigue and improves immunity

Suitable: green peppers + cauliflower = skin care

Avoid: green peppers + sunflower seeds = prevents the absorption of vitamin E

Avoid: green peppers + coriander = oxidizes the vitamin C

Cooking Tip
Dish up the green pepper after it is cooked, and season it with some vinegar to reduce the loss of vitamin C.

Healthy Recipes
Steamed Mushrooms with Green Peppers

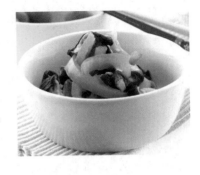

Ingredients: 150 g (5 oz) green pepper, 50 g (2 oz) water-swollen mushrooms, 20 g (1 oz) vegetable oil, 3 g (0.1 oz) each monosodium glutamate and salt, 500 g (18 oz) water

Preparation: ❶Remove the green pepper's seeds, then wash it and cut it into strips; cut the mushrooms into small cubes. ❷Dish up green pepper and mushroom cubes and add vegetable oil, salt and monosodium glutamate and stir evenly. ❸Pour water into the pot and bring to a boil. Lay green pepper and mushroom cubes on the steaming tray and wait for about 20 minutes until they are cooked.

Green Peppers and Shredded Tofu

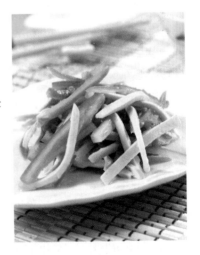

Ingredients: 250 g (9 oz) green peppers; 100 g (3.5 oz) thin sheets of bean curd; 2 g (0.1) each minced garlic, chopped green onion, Sichuan pepper powder, salt and monosodium glutamate; 15 g (0.5 oz) vegetable oil

Preparation: ❶Wash green peppers, remove their pedicles and seeds and cut it into shreds; wash the thin sheets of bean curd and cut into shreds. ❷Heat some vegetable oil in a pan; when the oil is 70 percent heated, add the chopped green onions and Sichuan pepper powder and stir-fry until fragrant; add green pepper and bean curd to stir-fry for five minutes; season with salt, minced garlic and monosodium glutamate.

Cucumber

Properties and taste: cool; sweet
Channels of entry: lung, spleen, stomach, bladder
Essentials of pharmacopoeia: As recorded in the *Compendium of Materia Medica*, the cucumber clears heat, quenches thirst and alleviates water retention. Frequent consumption is not suggested, as too much cucumber can cause chills and fever, damage yin-fluid and blood, and induce sores, beriberi and puffiness.

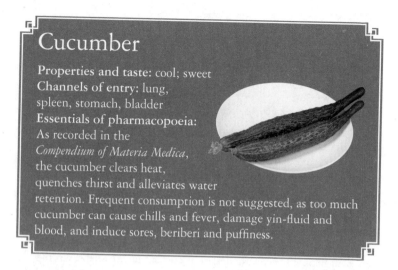

Health Effects

Protecting and nourishing the skin: Cucumbers contain a variety of vitamins and are rich in enzymes of biological activity, and they promote body metabolism. Cucumber juice can be applied to the skin for amazing cosmetic results such as moisturizing and wrinkle removal, so the cucumber is also known as the "skin care vegetable in the kitchen."

Anti-aging: Cucumber is rich in vitamin E, which prolongs life and provides anti-aging effects.

Strengthening physical fitness: The vitamin C in cucumber improves the body's immunity.

Points of Attention for Different People

Suitable for beauty pursuers: The cucumber's juice works to moisturize skin and remove wrinkles.

Suitable for patients with diabetes: Cucumbers prevent the saccharides from turning into fat.

Suitable for patients with hepatopathy: The cucumber contains amino acids essential to human body such as arginine, and it is quite helpful to the recovery of the patient with hepatopathy.

Food Compatibility and Incompatibility

Suitable: cucumbers + tomatoes = maintains the body's salt balance

Suitable: cucumbers + apples = promotes gastrointestinal peristalsis

Avoid: cucumbers + Chinese wolfberries = excessively high ratio of potassium

Eating Tip
It recommended that the cucumber seeds and peel are left intact because the cucumber is rich in carotene and the seeds are rich in vitamin E. In addition, the cucumber's pedicle is rich in bitter principle, a substance of anti-cancer effect, so do not throw it away.

Healthy Recipe
Cucumber and Shrimp Meat Soup
Ingredients: 100 g (3.5 oz) each cucumber and shrimp meat; 200 g (7 oz) bean curd; one egg; a little cooked sesame; 4 g (0.2 oz) salt; 2 g (0.1 oz) each white sugar, chopped scallion, rice wine, sesame oil, starch and fish soup-stock

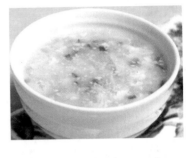

Preparation: ❶Whip the egg; wash and mince the shrimp, then add rice wine, chopped scallion, white sugar, sesame oil and salt to it and mix them up. Wash the bean curd and pound it with a pestle, and add salt, starch and whipped egg to it and mix. Wash and dice the cucumber. ❷Put fish soup-stock into the pot and add minced bean curd, shrimp mash and diced cucumber to the soup. Boil until the soup becomes thick, and season with salt and cooked sesame.

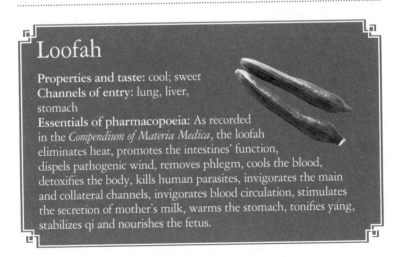

Loofah

Properties and taste: cool; sweet
Channels of entry: lung, liver, stomach
Essentials of pharmacopoeia: As recorded in the *Compendium of Materia Medica*, the loofah eliminates heat, promotes the intestines' function, dispels pathogenic wind, removes phlegm, cools the blood, detoxifies the body, kills human parasites, invigorates the main and collateral channels, invigorates blood circulation, stimulates the secretion of mother's milk, warms the stomach, tonifies yang, stabilizes qi and nourishes the fetus.

Health Effects

Clearing heat and detoxifying: Loofahs are sweet and cool in properties, and when eaten cooked or juiced they have functions such as clearing heat, removing phlegm, cooling the blood and detoxifying the body. They can also be used to treat diseases such as fever, polydipsia, cough, asthma due to excessive phlegm, hemafecia and hematuria.

Skin care: The loofah is rich in B vitamins that prevent skin aging and vitamin C that brightens skin, so it protects skin, dispels freckles and makes skin bright and delicate; loofah juice is called "beauty lotion."

Points of Attention for Different People

Suitable for people with constipation: The loofah doesn't contain many calories, and the phlegmatic temperament and saponin it contains are helpful to defecation.

Suitable for people with irregular menstruation: Frequent loofah consumption helps cure irregular menstruation.

Not suitable for people with deficiency-cold in the spleen and stomach, or diarrhea: The loofah is cool in properties, so it isn't suitable for these people.

Food Compatibility and Incompatibility

Suitable: loofahs + eggs = accelerates wound healing

Suitable: loofahs + shrimp = prevents and cures thyroid enlargement

Suitable: loofahs + coriander = reduces cancer morbidity

Avoid: loofahs + bamboo shoots = destroys carotinoid

Cooking Tip

If the loofah is fried with a thin peel, it will be juicy and crispy, but it may cause uncomfortable symptoms. Because the loofah is rich in mucilage and gelatinous fiber, if these substances are not cooked thoroughly, consumption stimulates the intestines and stomach, and the uncomfortable symptoms include loss of appetite, nausea caused by gastric disorder, chest distress or stomachache. Therefore, make sure that the loofah is well-cooked before eating it.

Healthy Recipes

Loofah and Sliced Meat Soup

Ingredients: 150 g (5 oz) lean pork; 75 g (3 oz) loofah; 10 g (0.4 oz) each vegetable oil and water; 2 g (0.1 oz) each chopped green onion, shredded ginger, pea starch, salt, monosodium glutamate, sesame oil and pepper

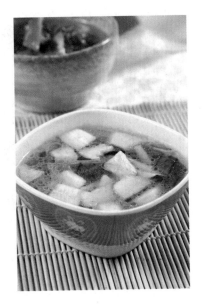

Preparation: ❶Wash and slice pork, and mix it evenly by adding starch, salt and water; peel, wash and dice the loofah. ❷Heat vegetable oil in a pot over medium heat, add the diced loofah, stir-fry it until it is 80 percent cooked and chewable; add boiled water to it and quick-boil the sliced meat when the soup boils. Sprinkle the soup with chopped green onion, shredded ginger, salt and monosodium glutamate; dish it up, season it with pepper and sprinkle the soup with sesame oil.

Tomatoes and Loofahs

Ingredients: 250 g (9 oz) loofahs; 100 g (3.5 oz) tomatoes; 2 g (0.1 oz) each chopped green onions, salt and monosodium glutamate; 10 g (0.4 oz) vegetable oil

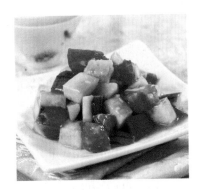

Preparation: ❶Peel, de-stem, wash and dice the loofahs and tomatoes. ❷Heat vegetable oil in a pan; add chopped green onion and stir-fry until fragrant, and when the oil is 70 percent cooked and a large amount of smoke comes from the pot, add diced loofah and tomato to the pan and stir-fry them until they are cooked; season with salt and monosodium glutamate to finish the dish.

Bitter Gourd

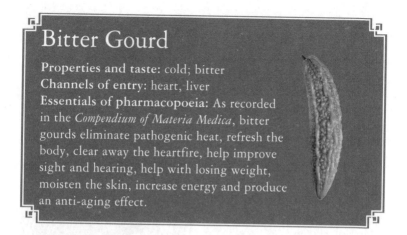

Properties and taste: cold; bitter
Channels of entry: heart, liver
Essentials of pharmacopoeia: As recorded in the *Compendium of Materia Medica*, bitter gourds eliminate pathogenic heat, refresh the body, clear away the heartfire, help improve sight and hearing, help with losing weight, moisten the skin, increase energy and produce an anti-aging effect.

Health Effects

Whetting the appetite: The bitter gourd contains charantin and bitter principle, which stimulate the appetite and tonify the spleen; it also contains quinine, which promotes urination, invigorates blood circulation, diminishes inflammation, brings down a fever, clears away the heart fire and improves eyesight.

Preventing and fighting cancer: Bitter gourds contain protein and a large amount of vitamin C, which enhances the body's immunologic function so the immune cells kills cancer cells.

Reducing blood glucose: The fresh juice of the bitter gourd contains charantin and substances similar to insulin, so it effectively reduces blood glucose and has a certain curative effect on diabetes.

Points of Attention for Different People

Suitable for patients with cancer: Bitter gourds improve the body's cancer-fighting ability.

Suitable for patients with diabetes: Bitter gourds help prevent and relieve the complications of diabetes.

Not suitable for pregnant women: Because bitter gourds contain quinine, which may cause spontaneous abortion, it is suggested that pregnant women avoid them.

Food Compatibility and Incompatibility

Suitable: bitter gourds + lean meat = enhances physical strength

Suitable: bitter gourds + asparagus = makes the skin look rosy

Avoid: bitter gourds + oysters = reduces nutritive value

Cooking Tip
It is suggested that the bitter gourd is stir-fried quickly over high heat or eaten uncooked and dressed with sauce. If the cooking time is too long, the water-soluble vitamins will be released and volatilized with the steam. As a result, the taste is affected, and nutrients are lost.

Healthy Recipes
Plain-Fried Bitter Gourds
Ingredients: 300 g (11 oz) bitter gourd; 2 g (0.1 oz) each salt, monosodium glutamate, white sugar and sesame oil; 10 g (0.4 oz) vegetable oil

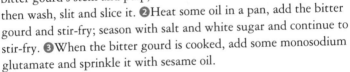

Preparation: ❶Remove the bitter gourd's stem and pulp, then wash, slit and slice it. ❷Heat some oil in a pan, add the bitter gourd and stir-fry; season with salt and white sugar and continue to stir-fry. ❸When the bitter gourd is cooked, add some monosodium glutamate and sprinkle it with sesame oil.

Bitter Gourd and Pork Ribs Soup
Ingredients: 250 g (9 oz) bitter gourd; 200 g (7 oz) pork ribs; 2 g (0.1 oz) each green onion strips, ginger slices, rice wine and salt; 500 g (18 oz) water

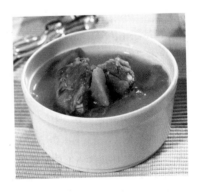

Preparation: ❶Remove bitter gourd's stem and pulp, then wash and dice it, and put it into boiling water for a few minutes; get it out and rinse it; wash the pork ribs and dice them. ❷Heat water in a pot and add the pork ribs. Adjust the heat to high and bring the water to a boil. After skimming off the foam, add green onion strips, ginger slices and rice wine to the soup; adjust the heat to the low and boil until the pork ribs are thoroughly cooked; add the bitter gourd to the soup and boil for another 10 minutes; season with salt to finish the dish.

White Gourd

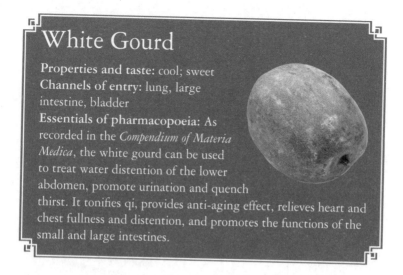

Properties and taste: cool; sweet
Channels of entry: lung, large intestine, bladder
Essentials of pharmacopoeia: As recorded in the *Compendium of Materia Medica*, the white gourd can be used to treat water distention of the lower abdomen, promote urination and quench thirst. It tonifies qi, provides anti-aging effect, relieves heart and chest fullness and distention, and promotes the functions of the small and large intestines.

Health Effects

Lowering blood pressure and alleviating water retention: White gourds are rich in protein, dietary fiber and a variety of mineral substances, and they are high in sylvite while low in sodium, so they provide good auxiliary dietary therapy for diseases such as arteriosclerosis, coronary heart disease, hypertension, edema and abdominal distension.

Lowering lipid and helping weight loss: The white gourd is characterized by low fat and low calories, and the tartronic acid it contains effectively inhibits saccharides from transforming into fat, so it is of great significance in avoiding weight gain; therefore, it is known as an "ideal food for weight control."

Points of Attention for Different People

Suitable for patients with hypertension: White gourds are high in potassium and low in sodium, so they are an ideal food for the patient with hypertension.

Suitable for obese people: The white gourd is rich in tartronic acid and it provides a good anti-obesity effect.

Not suitable for people with weak spleen and stomach: White gourds are cool in nature and it is suggested that these people should eat them less frequently.

Food Compatibility and Incompatibility
Suitable: white gourds + shrimp = helps the human body absorb calcium

Suitable: white gourds + duck = prevents anemia and improves appetite

Avoid: white gourds + pork liver = destroys vitamin C

Cooking Tip
White gourds are quite juicy, and if they aren't cooked immediately after they are purchased, do not peel them—it is best to wrap the white gourd with cling wrap, put it into a plastic bag and store in the refrigerator. It can be kept fresh for about one week, and massive loss of nutrients can be avoided.

Healthy Recipe
White Gourd, Pearl Barley and Duck Soup

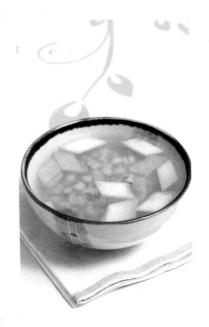

Ingredients: 100 g (3.5 oz) duck meat, 200 g (7 oz) white gourd, 50 g (2 oz) pearl barley, 3 g (0.1 oz) salt, 1 g (0.04 oz) monosodium glutamate, 2 g (0.1 oz) sesame oil, 50 g (2 oz) soup-stock

Preparation: ❶Wash and mince the duck meat; wash pearl barley and soak it for two hours; wash, peel and remove pulp of white gourd, and dice it. ❷Put soup-stock into a casserole pot and add the pearl barley; bring to a boil over high heat. ❸Adjust the heat to low and boil for another 30 minutes; add the white gourd to the soup and wait for 15 minutes until the gourd becomes tasty; add the minced duck meat to the soup and boil for several minutes. Finish the dish by seasoning it with salt and monosodium glutamate and sprinkling it with sesame oil.

Onion

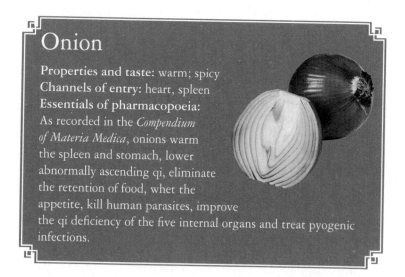

Properties and taste: warm; spicy
Channels of entry: heart, spleen
Essentials of pharmacopoeia:
As recorded in the *Compendium of Materia Medica*, onions warm the spleen and stomach, lower abnormally ascending qi, eliminate the retention of food, whet the appetite, kill human parasites, improve the qi deficiency of the five internal organs and treat pyogenic infections.

Health Effects

Whetting the appetite: The onion is spicy in flavor, and it stimulates the stomach, intestines and digestive gland secretions to whet the appetite.

Promoting digestion: The essential oil of onion contains sulfur compounds that reduce cholesterol, so it can be used to treat diseases such as anorexia and dyspepsia.

Reducing blood glucose and preventing cold: The onion helps cells to better utilize glucose and reduce blood glucose. Chewing fresh onion provides a sterilizing effect and prevents against cold.

Preventing and fighting cancer: The onion contains quercetin, which inhibits the growth of cancer cells; selenium, a micro-element, helps enhance cell viability and metabolism, and its functions also include cancer prevention and anti-aging.

Points of Attention for Different People

Suitable for patients with hypertension: Onions contain prostaglandin, and they promote the excretion of sodium and reduce blood pressure.

Suitable for patients with intestinal tract diseases: Onions contains phytocide with a special flavor, and it has antibacterial properties.

Not suitable for patients with skin disease: Eating onion causes excessive internal heat.

Food Compatibility and Incompatibility

Suitable: onions + pork = eliminates fatigue

Suitable: onions + pine nuts = anti-cancer, anti-aging and prevents heart disease

Suitable: onions + eggs = skin care and stimulates the blood circulation

Suitable: onions + beef = enhances immunity

Cooking Tip

Basically, onions can be divided into two types: onions with purple peels and onions with white peels, and the former contains more nutrients.

The white-peeled onion is quite tender, juicy and sweet. It looks golden and tastes very sweet if it is cooked for a long time, and it is recommended for eating raw. The purple-peeled onion has slightly red flesh and a strong, spicy flavor, and it is recommended for frying.

Healthy Recipe
Colored Peppers and Onion Rings

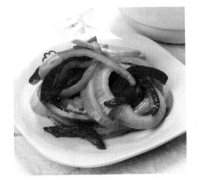

Ingredients: 300 g (11 oz) onions, 30 g (1 oz) each green pepper and cayenne pepper, 4 g (0.1 oz) salt, 15 g (0.5 oz) oil

Preparation: ❶ Wash onions and cut it into rings. ❷ Wash green peppers and cayenne peppers, remove their pedicles and seeds, and cut them into shreds. ❸ Heat some oil in a pan until it is about 50 percent heated, and put shredded peppers into the pan and stir-fry for several minutes. ❹ Put onion rings and salt into the pan and stir-fry them, and the dish is done when the color of onion rings changes slightly.

Cauliflower

Properties and taste: neutral; sweet
Channels of entry: spleen, stomach, kidney
Essentials of pharmacopoeia: As recorded in the *Compendium of Materia Medica*, long-term intake of cauliflower invigorates the kidneys, nourishes the brain, promotes the internal organs and the joints, improves eyesight and hearing, builds up strength, and strengthens muscles and bones.

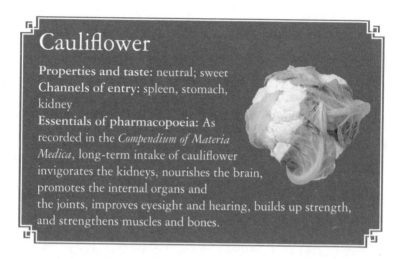

Health Effects

Preventing and fighting cancer: Cauliflower is rich in vitamin C, carotinoid and a variety of indole derivatives, and it improves the liver's ability to decompose cancerogenic substances and to some extent helps inhibit cytomorphosis of precancerous lesions and growth of cancer.

Cleaning blood vessel: Cauliflower is rich in flavonoids, which are the best vessel cleaner, as they prevent cholesterol from oxidizing and thrombocyte from coagulating; therefore, eating cauliflower reduces the risk of heart disease and stroke.

Points of Attention for Different People

Suitable for patients with cardiovascular disease: The flavonoids in cauliflower reduce the morbidity of cardiovascular disease.

Suitable for those with poor immunity: Cauliflower enhances the liver's detoxification capability and improves the body's immunity.

Food Compatibility and Incompatibility

Suitable: cauliflower + pork = skin whitening and enhances immunity

Suitable: cauliflower + shrimp = relieves thyroxine deficiency

Suitable: cauliflower + brown rice = skin care, cancer prevention and anti-aging

Avoid: cauliflower + pork liver = reduces the absorption rate of mineral substances

Cooking Tip

Although cauliflower is rich in nutrients, it contains pesticide residues and can have cabbageworms inside. Therefore, before eating it, soak it in saline water for several minutes to remove both the cabbageworms and pesticide residue.

Healthy Recipes

Cauliflower and Sliced Meat

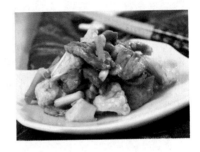

Ingredients: 300 g (11 oz) pork tenderloin; 200 g (7 oz) cauliflower; 15 g (0.5 oz) vegetable oil; 2 g (0.1 oz) each green onion strips, ginger slices, sweet sauce, soy sauce, dark soy sauce, zanthoxylum oil, rice wine, salt, monosodium glutamate, soup-stock, white sugar and starch

Preparation: ❶Wash and slice pork tenderloin, and season it with starch and dark soy sauce for later use; wash the cauliflower and break it off by hand into small pieces; scald it in boiling water and then drain it well for further use. ❷Heat oil in a pan, then add green onion strips and ginger slices and stir-fry them until fragrant; add sliced meat to the pan and stir-fry it until it is just cooked; add some sweet sauce, rice wine and soy sauce and stir-fry; add white sugar, monosodium glutamate, soup-stock and salt and stir-fry. ❸Put cauliflower into the pan and stir-fry it for three minutes, and sprinkle with zanthoxylum oil to serve.

Fried Ketchup and Cauliflower

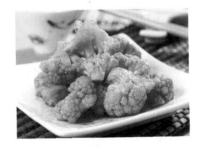

Ingredients: 500 g (18 oz) cauliflower; 2 g (0.1 oz) each ketchup, salt, monosodium glutamate; 15 g (0.5 oz) vegetable oil; 50 g (2 oz) water

Preparation: ❶Break cauliflower into small pieces and wash them; scald them in boiling water and drain well. ❷Heat oil in a pan, then add the cauliflower and water, and stir-fry for several minutes. ❸When the cauliflower is cooked, add ketchup, salt and monosodium glutamate.

Potato

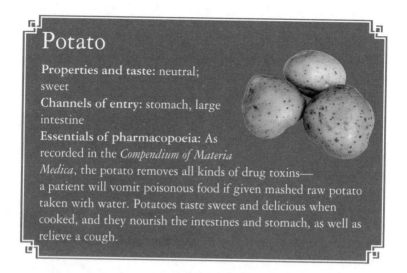

Properties and taste: neutral; sweet

Channels of entry: stomach, large intestine

Essentials of pharmacopoeia: As recorded in the *Compendium of Materia Medica*, the potato removes all kinds of drug toxins—a patient will vomit poisonous food if given mashed raw potato taken with water. Potatoes taste sweet and delicious when cooked, and they nourish the intestines and stomach, as well as relieve a cough.

Health Effects

Strengthening the spleen and nourishing the stomach: The potato is rich in starch, B vitamins, vitamin C and so on, and it promotes the digestion functions of the spleen and stomach.

Relaxing the intestine and bowel: The potato is rich in dietary fiber, and it relaxes the intestines and bowels; it also helps the human body to excrete and metabolize toxins to prevent constipation or diseases of the intestinal tract.

Points of Attention for Different People

Suitable for obese people: The potato is low in fat, and it can also help metabolize the body's excess fat.

Suitable for beauty pursuers: Potato juice applied to the face brightens the skin.

Not suitable for patients with asthma: Due to the aerogenesis, the potato will lead to abdominal distension.

Not suitable for people with stomachache or abdominal distension: Due to aerogenesis, the potato aggravates the abdominal distension and stomachache.

Food Compatibility and Incompatibility

Suitable: potatoes + eggs = moistens the skin and eliminates fatigue

Suitable: potatoes + pork = eliminates fatigue

Avoid: potatoes + taro = excessive intake of starch

Eating Tip

Unripe, sprouted or green potatoes are high in solanine, which is a toxic substance and will cause poisoning symptoms, so do not eat these kinds of potatoes.

Healthy Recipes
Sweet and Sour Shredded Potatoes

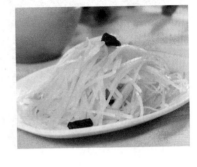

Ingredients: 500 g (18 oz) potatoes; 20 g (1 oz) vegetable oil; 2 g (0.1 oz) each vinegar, salt, green onion strips, Sichuan peppers, monosodium glutamate, dried pimiento

Preparation: ❶Wash, peel and shred the potatoes; soak in cold water for 10 minutes and drain well. ❷Heat some oil in a pan, then add Sichuan peppers; remove when they turn dark. ❸Add some dried pimiento to the oil, and then put the well-drained shredded potatoes into the pan immediately and stir-fry for a few minutes; add some vinegar and salt; when the shredded potatoes are almost cooked, add green onion strips and monosodium glutamate and mix evenly.

Potato and Spinach Soup

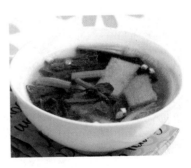

Ingredients: 200 g (7 oz) potato, 100 g (3.5 oz) spinach, 4 g (0.2 oz) salt, 3 g (0.1 oz) each vinegar and chopped scallion, 300 g (11 oz) water

Preparation: ❶Wash and slice the potato. Boil potatoes until they are 70 percent cooked and chewable, and then remove from the water. Wash and scald the spinach, and then cut it into strips. ❷Add sliced potatoes to the boiling water, and wait until the potatoes are cooked, then season with vinegar. Add the spinach strips to the soup and bring it to a boil; finish the dish by seasoning it with salt and chopped scallions.

Yam

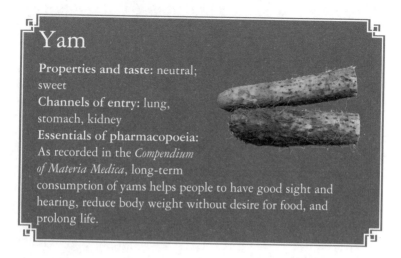

Properties and taste: neutral; sweet
Channels of entry: lung, stomach, kidney
Essentials of pharmacopoeia: As recorded in the *Compendium of Materia Medica*, long-term consumption of yams helps people to have good sight and hearing, reduce body weight without desire for food, and prolong life.

Health Effects

Nourishing and building up the body: Yams are rich in substances such as mucoprotein, amylase, free amino acids and polyphenol oxidase, so they are nourishing. Yams promote dietetic invigoration for rehabilitation after any illness.

Anti-obesity and weight loss: Yams have a high dietary fiber, choline and mucilage content, and effectively prevent fat deposition in the cardiovascular system and maintain vascular elasticity. Frequent yam consumption reduces the deposit of subcutaneous fat and helps prevent obesity.

Points of Attention for Different People

Suitable for obese people: Yams are an ideal food for bodybuilding. They prevent damage to the body during a diet and help obese people to lose weight if they're used as staple food.

Not suitable for people with constipation: Yams induce astringency, so it isn't suggested that those with constipation eat them.

Food Compatibility and Incompatibility

Suitable: yams + pork = brightens the skin and eliminates fatigue

Suitable: yams + duck meat = treats yin deficiency and tonifies the lungs

Suitable: yams + bitter gourds = weight loss and expulsion of toxins

Avoid: yams + carrots = destroys vitamin C

Avoid: yams + pineapples = hampers health of intestines and stomach

Cooking Tip

A long cooking period is not suggested for yams, because the amylase they contain will be destroyed if overcooked, and its functions such as tonifying the spleen and helping indigestion will be reduced; other nutrients will also be destroyed if yams are boiled too long.

Healthy Recipes

Yams in Hot Toffee

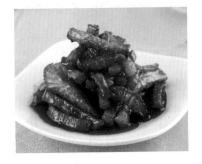

Ingredients: 260 g (9 oz) yams, 60 g (2 oz) cooked sesame powder, 2 g (0.1 oz) white sugar, 30 g (1 oz) vegetable oil

Preparation: ❶Wash and peel the yams and cut into strips 1 cm in width. ❷Heat oil in a pan over medium heat, and when the oil is about 50 percent heated, put the yam strips into the pan until they are deep fried, then remove them to a colander. ❸Leave some oil in the pan; put the white sugar into the pan and when the sugar juice becomes quite thick put the yams back in the pan; stir-fry the yams by flipping them over until evenly coated with sugar juice; sprinkle with cooked sesame powder and dish it up using a dish greased with oil.

Crystal Sugar and Yam Soup

Ingredients: 250 g (9 oz) yams, 10 g (0.4 oz) crystal sugar, 100 g (3.5 oz) water

Preparation: ❶Wash, peel and dice the yams. ❷Bring a pot of water to a boil and add the diced yams; when the yams are 60 percent cooked and chewable, add crystal sugar to the soup. The dish is done when the yams become soft and waxy and the sugar juice becomes thick.

Lotus Root

Properties and taste: cold; sweet
Channels of entry: heart, spleen, lung
Essentials of pharmacopoeia: As recorded in the *Compendium of Materia Medica*, the lotus root invigorates the spleen-stomach, helps people to attain mental tranquility, and cures numerous diseases. Frequent lotus root consumption reduces bodyweight, provides an anti-aging effect and prolongs life. Lotus roots dispel cold, remove dampness and relieve splenic diarrhea.

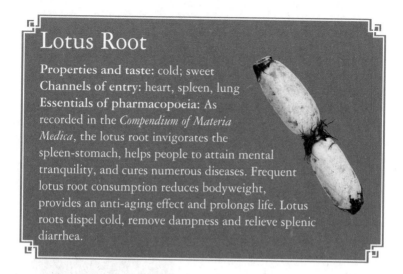

Health Effects

Clearing heat and cooling the blood: The lotus root is cold in properties, and it clears heat, cools blood and can be used to treat fever and inflammation.

Tonifying the spleen and stimulating appetite: The lotus root emits a special flavor, and it also contains tannins; it tonifies the spleen, provides antidiarrheic effects, whets the appetite and promotes digestion, so it helps those lacking an appetite to regain their health.

Stopping bleeding and dispersing blood stasis: The lotus root is rich in tannins, which are vasoconstrictive, so its functions include hemostasis. According to Chinese medicine, it promotes hemostasis without causing blood stagnation, so it provides ideal dietary therapy in treating a mass formed by blood stasis caused by heat disease.

Points of Attention for Different People

Suitable for patients with hemorrhagic disease: Lotus roots can promote hemostasis.

Suitable for patients with diabetes and hypertension: The dietary fiber in lotus roots promotes excretion of cholesterol and sugar and helps prevent diabetes and hypertension.

Not suitable for parturients: The lotus root is cold in properties, and it is not suggested that the parturient eat it immediately after delivery, but it helps clear stagnant blood if eaten one to two weeks post-delivery.

Food Compatibility and Incompatibility
Suitable: lotus roots + crystal sugar = tonifies the spleen, stimulates the appetite and stops diarrhea
  Suitable: lotus roots + mung beans = clears internal heat, cools down blood and reduces blood pressure
  Suitable: lotus roots + ginger = treats seasonal summer stomach and intestinal diseases

Cooking Tip
It is suggested that vessels made of ceramics or stainless steel be used if the lotus roots are stewed for a long time; reduce oxidation by avoiding cooking lotus roots in iron or aluminum pots, or cutting them with iron knives.

Healthy Recipe
Honeydew Lotus Roots
Ingredients: 500 g (18 oz) lotus roots, 10 g (0.4 oz) honey, 100 g (3.5 oz) water

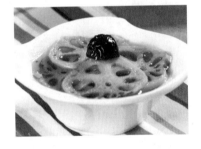

  Preparation: ❶Peel, wash and slice the lotus roots and then dish up. ❷Sprinkle the lotus root slices evenly with honey. ❸Put the lotus root slices sprinkled with honey into the steamer and steam for 15 minutes.

Bamboo Shoot

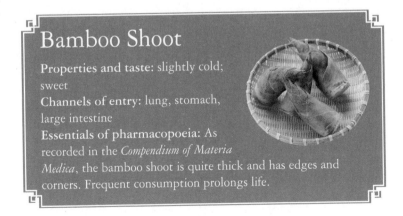

Properties and taste: slightly cold; sweet
Channels of entry: lung, stomach, large intestine
Essentials of pharmacopoeia: As recorded in the *Compendium of Materia Medica*, the bamboo shoot is quite thick and has edges and corners. Frequent consumption prolongs life.

Health Effects

Anti-obesity and weight loss: Bamboo shoots are rich in dietary fiber, B vitamins and nicotinic acid, and they absorb a large amount of greasy fat and reduce the absorption and accumulation of fat by the gastrointestinal mucosa, so they provide a good anti-obesity effect.

Helping digestion and relaxing the bowel: Bamboo shoots are rich in nicotinic acid and dietary fiber, which promote intestinal tract movement, help indigestion, eliminate food retention and prevent constipation, so they have some preventive effects on tumors in the digestive tract.

Points of Attention for Different People

Suitable for people with constipation: Bamboo shoots are rich in dietary fiber and they promote intestinal tract movement and prevent constipation.

Suitable for obese people: Bamboo shoots reduce absorption and accumulation of fat by the gastrointestinal mucosa.

Not suitable for patients with urticaria: They are allergenic.

Food Compatibility and Incompatibility

Suitable: bamboo shoots + eggs = maintains the health of the digestive system

Suitable: bamboo shoots + oysters = promotes wound healing and prevents the cold

Avoid: bamboo shoots + carrots = destroy carotinoid

Avoid: bamboo shoots + bean curd = reduces calcium absorption

Cooking Tip

Bamboo shoots are high in oxalic acid, and they produce an insoluble substance called calcium oxalate if they are taken with food containing calcium, thus affecting the body's calcium intake of calcium; meanwhile, high oxalic acid content induces or aggravates the symptoms of lithiasis. Therefore, before cooking, it is suggested that the bamboo shoots are quick-boiled to remove excessive oxalic acid.

Healthy Recipe

Fried Shredded Chicken with Bamboo Shoots

Ingredients: 250 g (9 oz) chicken breast; 100 g (2.5 oz) bamboo shoots; 30 g (1 oz) each green peppers and cayenne peppers; 5 g (0.2 oz) each green onion strips and ginger slices; 2 g (0.1 oz) each rice

wine, water starch, salt, soy sauce
and monosodium glutamate
    Preparation: ❶Wash
and shred the chicken breast,
season it with salt, rice wine,
soy sauce and water starch, and
mix it up evenly for further use.
❷Wash, shred and scald the
bamboo shoots; remove pedicles
and seeds of green and cayenne
peppers, and wash and shred them. ❸Heat some oil in a pan until it's
70 percent heated, stir-fry green onion strips and ginger slices until
fragrant, and put shredded chicken into the pan until it becomes
loose. ❹Add bamboo shoots, green and cayenne peppers and continue
to stir-fry; add some water and cover the pan with a lid. Stew until
almost cooked; season with salt and monosodium glutamate and stir-
fry evenly before dishing up.

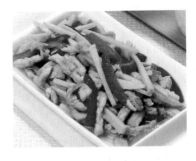

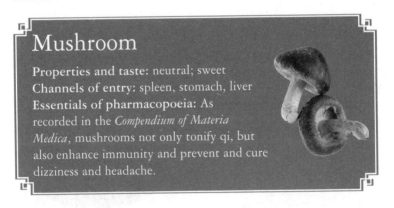

Mushroom

Properties and taste: neutral; sweet
Channels of entry: spleen, stomach, liver
Essentials of pharmacopoeia: As
recorded in the *Compendium of Materia
Medica*, mushrooms not only tonify qi, but
also enhance immunity and prevent and cure
dizziness and headache.

Health Effects

Supplementing vitamins: Mushrooms contain up to 18 kinds of
amino acids, and are also rich in glutamate and a variety of vitamins
and protein, so they are known as a "treasure-house of vitamins."

    Preventing cancer: The ribonucleic acid in mushrooms produces
anticancer interferons; polysaccharides contained in mushrooms
improve activity of anticancer immune cell in the human body, so
frequent mushroom consumption provides an anticancer effect.

Points of Attention for Different People

Suitable for cancer patients: Frequent mushroom consumption inhibits the growth of tumor cells.

Suitable for patients with hypertension: Mushrooms help reduce cholesterol and blood pressure.

Suitable for beauty pursuers: It strengthens the spleen and stomach functions, improves brain health, soothes the nerves, and protects and nourishes the skin if we eat mushrooms frequently.

Not suitable for people with itchy skin: The mushroom aggravates the symptoms.

Food Compatibility and Incompatibility

Suitable: mushrooms + celery = protects eyesight, offers anti-aging and cancer prevention

Suitable: mushrooms + lean meat = maintains the health of the digestive system

Suitable: mushrooms + bean curd = enhances anticancer function and reduces blood fat

Cooking Tip

It is suggested that dried mushrooms are soaked in water at 80 degrees Celsius (176 degrees Fahrenheit) until they are well-swollen, as then the mushrooms' ribonucleic acid can be catalyzed and the substances with delicate flavor will be released. However, do not soak them too long, in case the delicate flavors become lost.

Healthy Recipe

Mushrooms and Bamboo Shoots Soup

Ingredients: 200 g (7 oz) bamboo shoots, five pieces of dried mushrooms, 50 g (2 oz) Chinese cabbage hearts, 4 g (0.2 oz) salt, 2 g (0.1 oz) monosodium glutamate, a little sesame oil, 500 g (18 oz) water

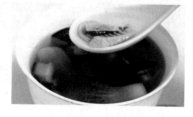

Preparation: ❶Soak the mushrooms in water until they are well-swollen, remove stems, and wash and cut every mushroom into four pieces. Shell and slice the bamboo shoots; wash the Chinese cabbage hearts and cut them into strips. ❷Put mushrooms and bamboo shoots into a pot and add water; bring to a boil. ❸Before dishing up, add some heart of Chinese cabbage to the soup and boil for a few minutes; then season the soup with salt and monosodium glutamate, and sprinkle it with a little sesame oil.

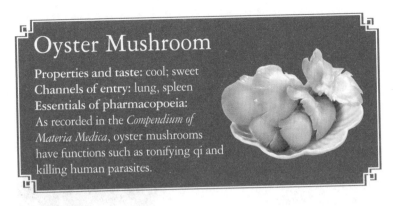

Oyster Mushroom

Properties and taste: cool; sweet
Channels of entry: lung, spleen
Essentials of pharmacopoeia:
As recorded in the *Compendium of Materia Medica*, oyster mushrooms have functions such as tonifying qi and killing human parasites.

Health Effects

Nourishing and building the body: The oyster mushroom is rich in a variety of vitamins and mineral substances, and it can be taken as nourishment for weak patients. It also has positive effects for those with hepatitis, chronic gastritis, stomach and duodenal ulcer, chondropathy and hypertension.

Sterilization and anti-tumor: Oyster mushrooms contain substances such as selenium and polysaccharide, and these effectively inhibits tumor cells. Pleurotus toxin and mushroom ribonic acid in oyster mushrooms inhibit the synthesis and reproduction of viruses.

Points of Attention for Different People

Suitable for cancer patients: The oyster mushroom is an anti-cancer food, and its anti-cancer and cancer preventive functions are quite direct.

Suitable for people with pain in the waist and legs: The functions of the oyster mushroom include relieving rheumatic pains, dispelling cold, stimulating blood circulation and relaxing muscles and joints.

Food Compatibility and Incompatibility

Suitable: oyster mushrooms + hotbed leeks = builds up body strength and promotes digestion

Suitable: oyster mushrooms + beef = cancer prevention, anti-cancer and enhances human immunity

Suitable: oyster mushrooms + pork = improves the body's metabolism

Eating Tip

There is viscous substance on the surface of oyster mushrooms, so wash before eating. For both dried and fresh oyster mushrooms, avoid prolonged soaking in water, as this would cause a massive loss of nutrients.

Healthy Recipe
Fried Oyster Mushrooms

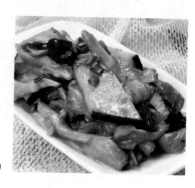

Ingredients: 250 g (9 oz) oyster mushrooms; 150 g (5 oz) cucumbers; 5 g (0.2 oz) each chopped green onion, shredded ginger and minced garlic; 8 g (0.3 oz) dried pimiento; 6 g (0.2 oz) each soy sauce and white sugar; 3 g (0.1 oz) salt; 2 g (0.1 oz) sesame oil; 20 g (1 oz) cooking oil

Preparation: ❶Trim and tear oyster mushrooms into small pieces and wash them piece by piece, then scald them in boiling water; tear the oyster mushrooms into strips after draining well and squeezing off the water; wash and slice the cucumbers. ❷Heat cooking oil in a pan, and when the oil is 50 percent heated, add chopped green onion, shredded ginger, minced garlic and dried pimiento to the pan, and stir-fry until fragrant. ❸Put the oyster mushroom strips into the pan and stir-fry for one minute; season with soy sauce, salt and white sugar and stir-fry for two more minutes; put the cucumber slices into the pan and continue to stir-fry for 20 seconds. Sprinkle with sesame oil before dishing up.

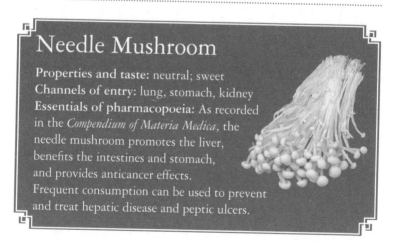

Needle Mushroom

Properties and taste: neutral; sweet
Channels of entry: lung, stomach, kidney
Essentials of pharmacopoeia: As recorded in the *Compendium of Materia Medica*, the needle mushroom promotes the liver, benefits the intestines and stomach, and provides anticancer effects.
Frequent consumption can be used to prevent and treat hepatic disease and peptic ulcers.

Health Effects
Decreasing blood pressure and blood fat: Needle mushrooms are high in potassium and low in sodium, and they are the ideal food for patients with hypertension, obese people and middle-aged and elderly people, as they inhibit the increase of blood fat levels, reduce cholesterol, and prevent and cure cardiovascular and cerebrovascular diseases.

Invigorating the brain and improving brain health: Needle mushrooms are rich in lysine and zinc, so they help children's brain development. It is known as the "mushroom that promote intelligence."

Points of Attention for Different People
Suitable for children: Needle mushrooms are high in zinc, which promotes children's intelligence development and invigorates their brains.

Suitable for cancer patients: Needle mushrooms contain a substance called flammulin, which enhances the human body's defense capability against cancer cells.

Not suitable for people with gout: Needle mushrooms generate a large amount of uric acid in the body and aggravate the symptoms of gout, so frequent intake is not suggested.

Food Compatibility and Incompatibility
Suitable: needle mushrooms + bean curd = improves brain health and builds up the body

Suitable: needle mushrooms + chicken = enriches the blood and tonifies qi

Suitable: needle mushrooms + cauliflower = enhances human immunity

Cooking Tip
Remove the root of needle mushrooms before cooking them. Fresh needle mushrooms contain colchicine, so too much uncooked mushroom can irritate the intestines, stomach and the respiratory tract's mucous membrane, with symptoms including nausea, vomiting, stomachache, diarrhea, or even fever and electrolyte disturbance. However, as long as the needle mushroom is well-cooked, the colchicine will be decomposed and destroyed.

Healthy Recipe
Garlicky Hot Green Peppers and
Needle Mushrooms

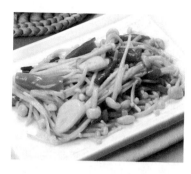

Ingredients: 200 g (7 oz) needle
mushrooms, 100 g (3.5 oz) hot
green peppers, 5 g (0.2 oz) sliced
garlic, 3 g (0.1 oz) salt, 2 g
(0.1 oz) monosodium glutamate

Preparation: ❶Remove the
roots of the needle mushrooms,
wash and tear the mushrooms into small pieces. ❷Remove the pedicle
and seeds of the hot green peppers, then wash and cut them into strips
about 2 cm in length. ❸Heat some oil in a pan, then add sliced garlic
and hot green pepper strips to the pan; stir-fry until fragrant. ❹Add
needle mushrooms, adjust the heat to high, and quick-fry evenly; when
the needle mushrooms become soft, season with salt and monosodium
glutamate and dish it up.

Black Fungus

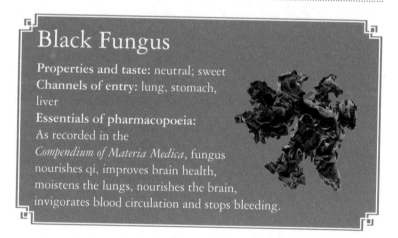

Properties and taste: neutral; sweet
Channels of entry: lung, stomach,
liver
Essentials of pharmacopoeia:
As recorded in the
Compendium of Materia Medica, fungus
nourishes qi, improves brain health,
moistens the lungs, nourishes the brain,
invigorates blood circulation and stops bleeding.

Health Effects

Enriching the blood and nourishing the skin: Black fungus is rich
in iron, which maintains beauty, keeps people young and prevents
anemia; it is rich in colloids, which help treat yin deficiency, moisturize
skin and promote excretion.

Preventing thrombus: Black fungus contains vitamin K, which reduces blood clotting, prevents thrombus and so on; the phospholipid composition of black fungus decomposes cholesterol and triacylglycerol and promotes smooth blood circulation.

Points of Attention for Different People

Suitable for people with dyspepsia: Black fungus is rich in colloids, which clear and nourish the digestive system.

Suitable for cancer patients: The polysaccharide in black fungus increases the body's resistance tumors.

Food Compatibility and Incompatibility

Suitable: black fungus + eggs = strengthens the bones and teeth

Suitable: black fungus + shrimp = brightens the skin and nourishes the hair

Suitable: black fungus + red dates = strengthens the spleen and stomach functions and enriches the blood

Cooking Tip

The fresh black fungus contains photoactive substances; people will have symptoms such as pruritus, pain and edema of the skin when exposed to strong sunlight after eating fresh black fungus. Most of photoactive substances are eliminated in the dried black fungus after exposure to strong sunlight and being soaked in water.

Healthy Recipe

Fried Green Peppers and Fungus

Ingredients: 200 g (7 oz) water-swollen fungus, 100 g (3.5 oz) carrots, 80 g (3 oz) green peppers, 5 g (0.2 oz) each sliced scallions and shredded ginger, 3 g (0.1 oz) salt, 2 g (0.1 oz) monosodium glutamate, 10 g (0.4 oz) water

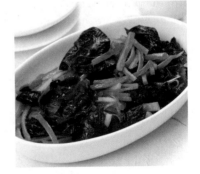

Preparation: ❶ Remove stems from black fungus, wash fungus and tear into small pieces. ❷Wash and shred the carrots; wash, remove pedicle and seeds of green peppers and shed them. ❸Heat some oil in a pan, then stir-fry the sliced scallions and shredded ginger until fragrant. ❹Put black fungus, carrots and green peppers into the pan and stir-fry them; add salt and water, and stir-fry until cooked. Season with monosodium glutamate to serve.

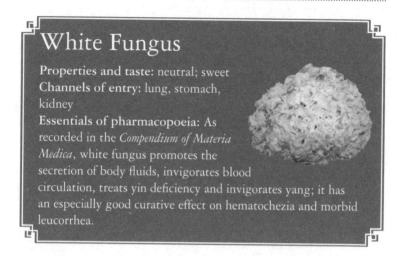

White Fungus

Properties and taste: neutral; sweet
Channels of entry: lung, stomach, kidney
Essentials of pharmacopoeia: As recorded in the *Compendium of Materia Medica*, white fungus promotes the secretion of body fluids, invigorates blood circulation, treats yin deficiency and invigorates yang; it has an especially good curative effect on hematochezia and morbid leucorrhea.

Health Effects

Improving complexion and reducing weight: White fungus is rich in natural plant gum, which can be used to treat yin deficiency, nourish the skin, purge the intestines and regulate the stomach, and long-term consumption of white fungus dispels chloasma and freckles. White fungus is rich in dietary fiber, and it helps gastrointestinal peristalsis and reduces fat absorption.

Preventing osteoporosis: White fungus is rich in vitamin D, which prevents the calcium loss that would cause senile osteoporosis.

Detoxification and anti-tumor properties: White fungus is rich in microelements such as selenium, and it improves the liver's detoxification capability, enhances the body's ability to fight tumors, and it also boosts cancer patients' tolerance for radiotherapy and chemotherapy.

Points of Attention for Different People

Suitable for beauty pursuers: Long-term consumption of white fungus helps maintain the skin's moisture, and its functions also include dispelling chloasma and freckles.

Suitable for cancer patient: White fungus enhances the body's ability to resist tumors.

Food Compatibility and Incompatibility

Suitable: white fungus + lotus seeds = assists weight loss and dispels freckles

Suitable: white fungus + black fungus = moistens the lungs, enriches the blood and tonifies qi

Suitable: white fungus + squid = offers anti-cancer and anti-aging properties

Cooking Tip

The cooked white fungus of the previous night is not edible. White fungus is rich in nitrates, which will be restored to nitrite through bacteria decomposition if the fungus is stored for a long time after it is cooked. It is possible that the nitrite further transforms into nitrosamines, a cancerogenic substance.

Healthy Recipe
White Fungus, Papaya and Pork Ribs Soup

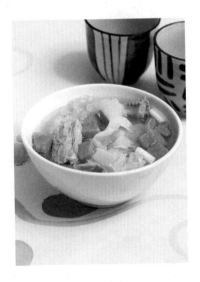

Ingredients: 250 g (9 oz) pork ribs, 5 g (0.2 oz) dried white fungus, 100 g (3.5 oz) papaya, 4 g (0.1 oz) salt, 3 g (0.1 oz) each green onion strips and ginger slices, 500 g (18 oz) water

Preparation: ❶Soak white fungus in water until it is well-swollen, then wash and tear it into small pieces; peel the papaya, remove its seeds and dice it; wash and dissect pork ribs, and scald them. ❷Pour water into a stockpot; add pork ribs, green onion strips and ginger slices to the water and boil them; add white fungus to the soup when the soup comes to a boil over high heat; adjust the heat to low and stew it for about an hour. ❸Add papaya to the soup and stew for 15 minutes; season with salt and dish it up.

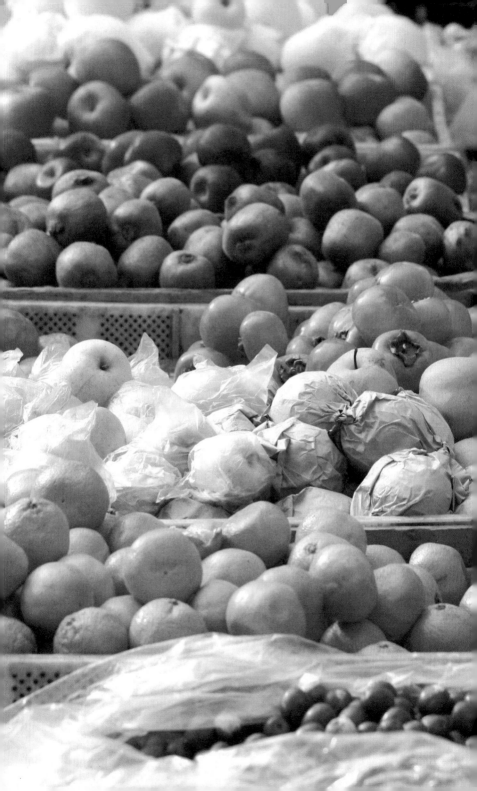

Chapter Four
Fruits and Nuts

Fruit is rich in vitamins, minerals and water, with health effects such as nourishing the skin, reducing weight and slimming the body, and preventing constipation. It can be eaten directly, and can also be used for cold salad, juice, etc. Nuts are often eaten as healthy snacks, and can also be used for cooking, making porridge, stewing soups, and more.

Banana

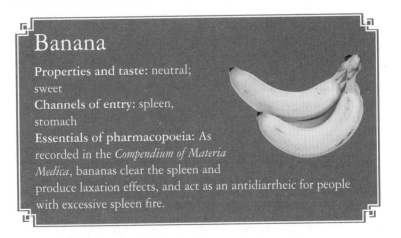

Properties and taste: neutral; sweet

Channels of entry: spleen, stomach

Essentials of pharmacopoeia: As recorded in the *Compendium of Materia Medica*, bananas clear the spleen and produce laxation effects, and act as an antidiarrheic for people with excessive spleen fire.

Health Effects

Lowering blood pressure and blood fat: Bananas are a fruit that can be taken both as medicine and food, as they are rich in a variety of vitamins. Bananas are high in potassium and low in sodium and cholesterol. Frequent banana consumption can effectively prevent and cure vascular sclerosis, reduce cholesterol, and prevent hypertension and high blood lipids.

Nourishing the stomach: Bananas contain a chemical substance that enhances protection of the gastric wall, helping prevent and cure stomach ulcers.

Sterilization and skin care: Bananas contain musarin, which inhibits the growth of fungi and bacteria, and they produce a good curative effect on tinea manuum and tinea corporis. Applying banana juice to the hands and face prevents skin aging, desquamation, pruritus and rhagades.

Replenishing energy: Bananas are high in potassium and sugar, so they provide immediate energy replenishment and protect myocardium; therefore, it is suggested that people eat them after exercising.

Points of Attention for Different People
Suitable for people with constipation: The banana's functions include lubricating the intestine and relaxing the bowel.

Not suitable for patients with diabetes: Bananas have a high sugar content.

Food Compatibility and Incompatibility
Suitable: bananas + cheese = prevents osteoporosis

Suitable: bananas + peanuts = improves the content of nicotinic acid

Suitable: bananas + white fungus = treats yin deficiency and moistens dryness

Avoid: bananas + potatoes = causes freckles on the face

Eating Tip
Do not eat too many bananas on an empty stomach in case the content of magnesium in the blood increases dramatically and inhibits the normal function of angiocarpy. The banana is high in potassium, so excessive intake of it will increase the blood potassium concentration, which is especially harmful for those with acute nephritis, chronic nephritis or renal insufficiency.

Healthy Recipes
Banana and Crystal Sugar Soup
Ingredients: One banana, 3 g (0.1 oz) each dried orange peel and crystal sugar, 300 g (11 oz) water

Preparation: ❶Peel the banana and cut it into chunks. ❷Soak the dried orange peel in warm water and wash it with clean water; shred it and put it into a pottery pot; pour 300 g water into the pot and bring it to a boil over high heat. ❸Add banana chunks to the pot, and when it boils, adjust the heat to low and continue to stew for 15 minutes; add crystal sugar and boil until the crystal sugar is dissolved; dish up.

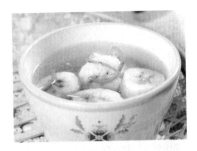

Stewed Bananas with Lily Bulbs

Ingredients: 15 g (0.5 oz) lily bulbs, two bananas, 3 g (0.1 oz) crystal sugar, 200 g (7 oz) water

Preparation: Peel and dice the bananas, then put all the ingredients into a pot and stew them until they look like porridge; the stew is done.

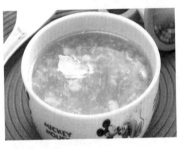

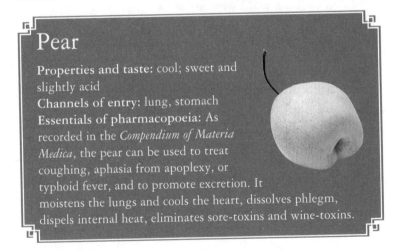

Pear

Properties and taste: cool; sweet and slightly acid

Channels of entry: lung, stomach

Essentials of pharmacopoeia: As recorded in the *Compendium of Materia Medica*, the pear can be used to treat coughing, aphasia from apoplexy, or typhoid fever, and to promote excretion. It moistens the lungs and cools the heart, dissolves phlegm, dispels internal heat, eliminates sore-toxins and wine-toxins.

Health Effects

Clearing away heart fire and moistening the lung: Eating pears frequently produces a curative effect on patients with pulmonary tuberculosis, tracheitis and upper respiratory infections.

Clearing internal heat and lowering blood pressure: Pears produce an anti-hypertensive effect and clear heat; frequent pear consumption is quite good for patients with hypertension, heart disease, hepatitis and liver cirrhosis.

Relieving autumn-dryness disease: It is quite dry in autumn, and people often experience itchy skin and a dry mouth and nose. Sometimes, they have dry cough with little phlegm; eating one pear a day helps relieve autumn-dryness disease and promotes health.

Points of Attention for Different People

Suitable for middle-aged and elderly people: Frequent pear consumption reduces blood pressure and prevents rheumatism and arthritis.

Suitable for pregnant women: Pears help relieve symptoms such as vomiting during the gestation period. However, pregnant women with a heightened miscarriage risk should not eat pears.

Not suitable for people with weak spleen and stomach functions: The pear is cool in properties, and excessive intake hurts the spleen and stomach.

Food Compatibility and Incompatibility

Suitable: pears + white fungus = treats yin deficiency, moistens dryness and eliminates lung fire

Suitable: pears + crystal sugar = moistens the lungs and relieves coughing

Suitable: pears + oranges = moisturizes and brightens the skin

Avoid: pears + sweet potatoes = induces gastrointestinal discomfort

Avoid: pears + mutton = causes dyspepsia

Eating Tip

It is suggested that people should limit themselves to one pear every day and try not to eat too much, as excessive intake will damage the spleen and stomach. In addition, do not drink too much water after eating pears, as it may cause diarrhea.

Healthy Recipes

Spinach and Pear Juice

Ingredients: 100 g (3.5 oz) spinach, 150 g (5 oz) pear, 2 g (0.1 oz) honey, 50 g (2 oz) drinking water

Preparation: ❶Wash and scald the spinach, soak it in cold water then drain; cut it into small strips; wash, core and dice the pear.

❷Put the above ingredients into a juicer, add drinking water for whipping, and then add the honey. Mix evenly and serve.

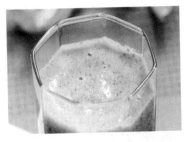

White Fungus and Pear Soup

Ingredients: 50 g (2 oz) white fungus; one pear; 10 g (0.4 oz) almonds; 150 g (5 oz) carrots; 2 g (0.1 oz) each dried orange peel, preserved dates and Chinese wolfberries; 500 g (18 oz) water

Preparation: ❶Soak white fungus in water until it is well-swollen, remove its yellow pedicle and tear the fungus into small pieces; wash, peel, core and dice the pear; wash the almonds;

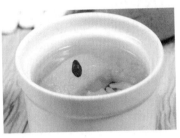

wash and dice the carrots. ❷Bring water and dried orange peel to a boil in a pot, then add the white fungus, diced pears, almonds, Chinese wolfberries, preserved dates and diced carrots, and boil over high heat for 20 minutes; adjust the heat to low and continue to stew for about three hours before dishing up.

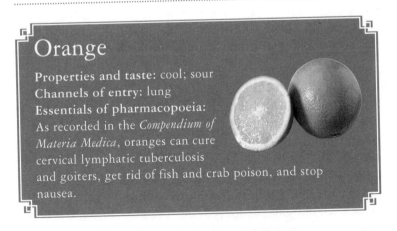

Orange

Properties and taste: cool; sour
Channels of entry: lung
Essentials of pharmacopoeia:
As recorded in the *Compendium of Materia Medica*, oranges can cure cervical lymphatic tuberculosis and goiters, get rid of fish and crab poison, and stop nausea.

Health Effects

Reducing blood fat and blood pressure: Oranges are rich in vitamin

C, which can increase the body's resistance, enhance the elasticity of capillaries, and reduce cholesterol in the blood. They are also good for hyperlipidemia, hypertension and arteriosclerosis.

Clearing and relaxing the bowels: Oranges' cellulose and pectin content can promote intestinal peristalsis, and oranges are conducive to bowel movements and eliminating harmful substances from the body.

Sterilizing and dispelling the effects of alcohol: Oranges are sour and fragrant. Acid can sterilize, harmonize the stomach, and calm the abnormal rise of qi. Oranges have good flavoring and detoxification effects for those who drink too much alcohol and are good to use when making fish and crab dishes.

Points of Attention for Different People

Suitable for heart-disease patients: Eating more oranges can increase the high-density lipoprotein levels in the body and reduce the risk of heart disease.

Suitable for women: The aroma of oranges helps women overcome tension.

Not suitable for people with indigestion: Organic acids in oranges can irritate the gastric mucosa, which is unfavorable to the stomach. People with indigestion should not eat them. Oranges are also not suitable for eating before meals or on an empty stomach.

Food Compatibility and Incompatibility

Suitable: oranges + mayonnaise = offers skin care, anti-cancer, anti-aging effects

Suitable: oranges + cream = reduces cholesterol absorption

Avoid: oranges + shrimp = produces indigestible substances

Avoid: oranges + pork = produces indigestible substances

Avoid: oranges + milk = affects protein absorption

Eating Tip

Immature oranges contain more oxalic acid, benzoic acid, etc., which can be easily combined with proteins in food to produce indigestible precipitates, thus affecting the body's protein absorption, and even lead to indigestion. Therefore, it is better not to eat immature oranges.

Healthy Recipes
Sweet Orange Juice
Ingredients: 250 g (9 oz) oranges; 3 g (0.1 oz) each ice cubes, lemon juice and white sugar; 100 g (3.5 oz) water

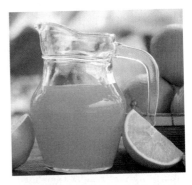

Preparation: ❶Wash the oranges, peel and cut them into pieces. ❷Put the chopped oranges into a juicer and add drinking water to whip them into juice. Add ice cubes, lemon juice and sugar.

White Turnip and Sweet Orange Juice
Ingredients: 100 g (3.5 oz) white turnips, 150 g (5 oz) oranges, 100 g (3.5 oz) drinking water

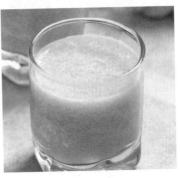

Preparation: ❶Wash white turnips, peel and dice them; peel and dice oranges. ❷Put the ingredients into a juicer and add 100 g drinking water for whipping.

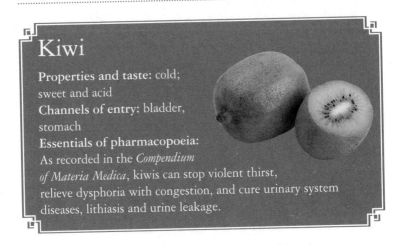

Kiwi

Properties and taste: cold; sweet and acid
Channels of entry: bladder, stomach
Essentials of pharmacopoeia:
As recorded in the *Compendium of Materia Medica*, kiwis can stop violent thirst, relieve dysphoria with congestion, and cure urinary system diseases, lithiasis and urine leakage.

Health Effects

Helping digestion and preventing constipation: Kiwis are rich in dietary fiber, which can not only reduce cholesterol and promote heart health, but also help digestion, prevent constipation and quickly remove harmful metabolites accumulated in the body.

Fighting cancer: The kiwi, known as the "king of vitamin C," has a good anti-oxidation effects, and can effectively block the formation of carcinogenic nitrosamines in the body. Therefore, it is useful to eat a kiwi after eating barbecued food and other cancerogenic food.

Beautification and weight-reduction: Kiwis are rich in vitamins E and K, and they have unique effects on bodybuilding and beautification. They contain folic acid, which can prevent fetal neural tube defects. Kiwi can also stimulate the accumulation of rich lutein on the retinas to prevent spots from getting worse.

Points of Attention for Different People

Suitable for elderly people: Kiwis can reduce cholesterol and produce an anti-cancer effect.

Suitable for women: Kiwis contain inositol, which helps to alleviate the tendency of depression during women's menstrual periods and childbirth.

Not suitable for people with weak spleen and stomach functions: These people should not eat much kiwi as it is cold in properties.

Food Compatibility and Incompatibility

Suitable: kiwis + pine nuts = promotes the body's iron absorption

Suitable: kiwis + mayonnaise = nourishes the skin and beautifies the complexion

Avoid: kiwis + pork = reduces nutritional value

Avoid: kiwis + cucumbers = destroys vitamin C

Eating Tip

The effect of eating a kiwi before a meal is different from the effect of eating one after. Eating kiwi before a meal mainly helps the body take in nutrients, while eating it after a meal can promote digestion.

Healthy Recipes

Celery-Kiwi Juice

Ingredients: 50 g (2 oz) celery, 150g (5 oz) kiwi, 2 g (0.1 oz) honey, 100 g (3.5 oz) drinking water

Preparation: ❶Wash the celery, remove the leaves, and cut it into small segments; peel and dice kiwi. ❷Put the above ingredients into a juicer, add drinking water for whipping, and then add the honey.

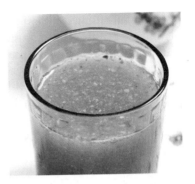

Cucumber-Kiwi Juice
Ingredients: 100 g (3.5 oz) cucumbers, 150 g (5 oz) grapefruit, 50 g (2 oz) each kiwi and lemon

Preparation: ❶Wash the cucumbers, cut them into small pieces; wash and peel the kiwi, cut it into small pieces; peel the grapefruit and lemon, and cut them into small pieces. ❷Put the above materials together with 50 g (2 oz) drinking water into a juicer for whipping.

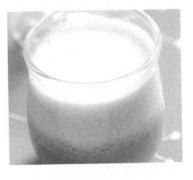

Cherry

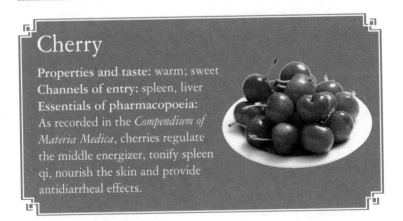

Properties and taste: warm; sweet
Channels of entry: spleen, liver
Essentials of pharmacopoeia:
As recorded in the *Compendium of Materia Medica*, cherries regulate the middle energizer, tonify spleen qi, nourish the skin and provide antidiarrheal effects.

Health Effects
Preventing eye disease: The cherry is rich in vitamin A, and frequent intake enhances eyesight. Cherries are also beneficial to the treatment of eye diseases, and prevent and cure nyctalopia and shortsightedness.

Supplementing iron and preventing anemia: The cherry is rich in iron, and frequent cherry consumption supplements the body's iron and promotes regeneration of hemoglobin. Cherries can be used to prevent and cure iron-deficiency anemia, strengthen physical fitness, invigorate the brain and improve brain health.

Protecting and nourishing the skin: The cherry is an excellent beauty food, as it is rich in carotene and vitamin C, and frequent cherry intake nourishes the skin and provides an anti-aging effect; it makes skin smooth, tender and rosy, dispelling wrinkles and freckles.

Points of Attention for Different People

Suitable for beauty pursuers: Cherry's functions include reducing wrinkles, dispelling freckles, and protecting and nourishing the skin.

Suitable for children: Frequent cherry consumption can supplement the body's iron levels and prevent iron-deficiency anemia.

Not suitable for people with constipation: Eating cherries can cause excessive internal heat and dry feces for these people.

Food Compatibility and Incompatibility

Suitable: cherries + cantaloupes = prevents anemia and builds up body strength

Suitable: cherries + salt = maintains acid-base equilibrium

Avoid: cherries + nut = tends to cause varicosity and blood stasis

Avoid: cherries + honey = reduces nutritive value

Eating Tip

Cherries are berries, which are perishable, so they are best preserved at -1 degree Celsius (about 30 degrees Fahrenheit). Do not wash cherries for a long time or soak them in water to avoid making their peels decay or their color change.

Healthy Recipes
Cherry Juice

Ingredients: 200 g (7 oz) cherries, 50 g (2 oz) drinking water

Preparation: ❶Wash, remove stems, halve and core cherries. ❷Put them into the juicer,

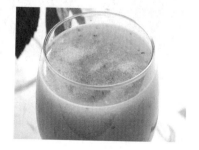

and add drinking water; it is done when they are whipped evenly.

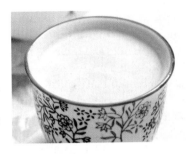

Cherry Yogurt

Ingredients: 200 g (7 oz) cherries, 300 ml (10 oz) yogurt

   Preparation: ❶Wash, remove stems, halve and core the cherries. ❷Put cherries and yogurt into the juicer and whip them evenly; the drink is done.

Grape

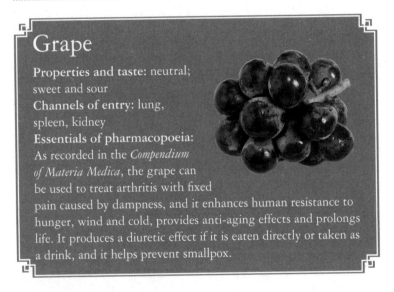

Properties and taste: neutral; sweet and sour

Channels of entry: lung, spleen, kidney

Essentials of pharmacopoeia: As recorded in the *Compendium of Materia Medica*, the grape can be used to treat arthritis with fixed pain caused by dampness, and it enhances human resistance to hunger, wind and cold, provides anti-aging effects and prolongs life. It produces a diuretic effect if it is eaten directly or taken as a drink, and it helps prevent smallpox.

Health Effects

Providing quick supplementation of glucose: The sugar that the grape contains is mainly glucose, which can be quickly absorbed by the body, so it helps prevent low blood glucose.

   Protecting blood vessel: The grape stops thrombosis and reduces the body's serum cholesterol levels, and to some extent, it helps prevent cardio-cerebrovascular diseases.

   Skin-care and anti-aging: The flesh of the grape is rich in nicotinic acid and mineral substances, and it effectively moisturizes the skin, promotes the reproduction of skin cells and provides anti-aging effects.

Points of Attention for Different People

Suitable for children and women: The raisin (dried grape) is rich in sugar and iron, and it can be taken as a tonic.

Suitable for cancer patients: The grape contains an effective anticancer substance and it prevents cancer cells from spreading.

Not suitable for patients with diabetes: Grapes are high in sugar, so it is not suggested that patients with diabetes eat them.

Food Compatibility and Incompatibility

Suitable: grapes + sesame = enhances effects of antioxidants

Suitable: grapes + glutinous rice = prevents anemia and eliminates fatigue

Avoid: grapes + radishes = inhibits the body's iodine absorption

Avoid: grapes + shrimp = causes stomach discomfort

Eating Tip

A daily intake of 10 to 13 grapes is suggested. As the old saying goes, "Spit no grape peels while eating grapes," which is reasonable, as most of the grape's nutrients are stored in the peels, and if people only eat the flesh, they lose many nutrients.

Healthy Recipes

Grape Yogurt

Ingredients: 250 g (9 oz) grapes, 300 ml (10 oz) yogurt, 2 g (0.1 oz) honey (optional)

Preparation: ❶Wash and halve the grapes and remove their seeds. ❷Put grapes and yogurt into the juicer and whip them evenly; finish the drink by seasoning it with honey.

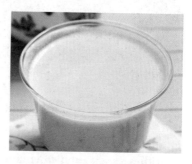

Tomato, Grape and Apple Drink

Ingredients: 200 g (7 oz) tomatoes, 100 g (3.5 oz) each grapes and apples, 10 g (0.4 oz) lemon juice, 100 g (3.5 oz) drinking water

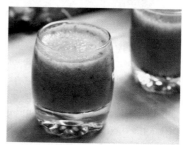

Preparation: ❶Wash and dice the tomatoes; wash grapes and remove seeds; wash, core and dice apples. ❷Put the above ingredients into a juicer, and add drinking water for whipping; pour the whipped juice into a glass and add some lemon juice to it.

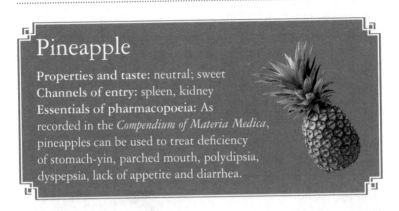

Pineapple

Properties and taste: neutral; sweet
Channels of entry: spleen, kidney
Essentials of pharmacopoeia: As recorded in the *Compendium of Materia Medica*, pineapples can be used to treat deficiency of stomach-yin, parched mouth, polydipsia, dyspepsia, lack of appetite and diarrhea.

Health Effects

Anti-thrombus: The pineapple contains bromelain, which accelerates the dissolution of fibrous protein and protein clots and reduces blood viscosity; it provides adjuvant therapy for cardiovascular and cerebrovascular diseases thanks to its anti-thrombus function.

Anti-inflammatory effects and easing swelling: Bromelain helps enhance local blood circulation, eliminate inflammation and edema, and accelerate tissue healing and repair.

Clearing heat and quenching thirst: Pineapples are rich in vitamin C, carbohydrates, moisture and all kinds of organic acids, and they clear summer-heat, tonify the spleen to quench thirst, dispel the effects of alcohol, and tonify qi.

Points of Attention for Different People

Suitable for patients with nephritis and hypertension: The pineapple has a diuretic function, and it is beneficial to the treatment of nephritis and hypertension if it is properly consumed.

Suitable for patients with coronary heart disease: The pineapple helps relieve heart disease caused by vascular thrombosis of the coronary and cerebral arteries.

Not suitable for people of allergic constitution: The pineapple is apt to cause an allergic reaction.

Food Compatibility and Incompatibility

Suitable: pineapples + pork = promotes the absorption of protein in pork

Suitable: pineapples + eggs = whitens the skin and eliminates fatigue

Avoid: pineapples + shrimp = stimulates the stomach and induces vomiting

Avoid: pineapples + bananas = high potassium content

Eating Tip

Do not eat too many pineapples, or else it stimulates the oral mucosa and weakens the sense of taste. Those who are allergic to bromelain will have symptoms such as itchy skin after eating pineapple; please seek medical advice as soon as possible if any allergic symptoms such as dizziness, vomiting, diarrhea, itching all over the body and redness on the skin appear after eating pineapple.

Healthy Recipes

Pineapple and Soy Milk Juice

Ingredients: 200 g (7 oz) pineapple (peeled), 300 ml (10 oz) soy milk

Preparation: ❶Dice the pineapple flesh and soak in light saline for about five minutes; remove and wash quickly. ❷Put pineapple and soy milk into the juicer and whip them.

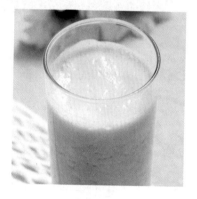

Kiwi, Pineapple and Apple Juice

Ingredients: 100 g (3.5 oz) each kiwi, apple and peeled pineapple

Preparation: ❶Wash and peel the kiwi, and dice the flesh; wash, peel, core and dice the apple; dice the pineapple and soak it in light saline for about 15 minutes; remove and wash quickly. ❷Put the above ingredients into a juicer and add 100 g (3.5 oz) drinking water for whipping.

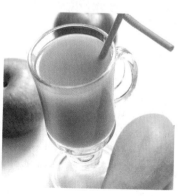

Papaya

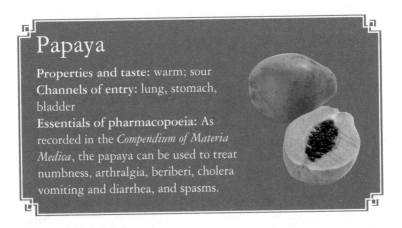

Properties and taste: warm; sour
Channels of entry: lung, stomach, bladder
Essentials of pharmacopoeia: As recorded in the *Compendium of Materia Medica*, the papaya can be used to treat numbness, arthralgia, beriberi, cholera vomiting and diarrhea, and spasms.

Health Effects

Tonifying the spleen and helping digestion: The papain in papaya can decompose fat into fatty acid and decomposes protein, so papaya is helpful for digestion and food absorption.

Promoting lactation: The chymosin in papaya promotes lactation.

Fighting cancer: The functions of carpaine include resistance against lymphatic leukemia, so papaya can be used to treat leukemia.

Antispasm: The papaya flesh contains carpaine, which helps relieve pain caused by spasms.

Points of Attention for Different People

Suitable for obese people: Papaya tonifies the spleen and helps digestion.

Suitable for the beauty pursuers: The functions of papaya include complexion improvement, weight reduction and breast enlargement.

Not suitable for people of allergic constitution: The carpaine in papaya is slightly toxic to the human body, so it isn't suggested that the people of allergic constitution eat it.

Not suitable for pregnant women: It induces uterine contractions.

Food Compatibility and Incompatibility

Suitable: papayas + milk = helpful for protein absorption

Suitable: papayas + pork = helpful for protein absorption

Avoid: papayas + pumpkins = reduces the nutritive value of papaya

Avoid: papayas + pork liver = destroys vitamin C of papaya

Eating Tip

The unripe papaya is high in phytoestrogen, so excessive intake could cause hormone imbalance.

Healthy Recipe

Stewed Papayas and Milk

Ingredients: 300 g (11 oz) papayas, 250 g (9 oz) milk, 80 g (3 oz) egg whites, 2 g (0.1 oz) each crystal sugar and vinegar

    Preparation: ❶Wash and halve the papayas and scoop out the insides with a spoon; put them into the juicer and puree. ❷Heat the milk in a pot, and when the milk boils, add the crystal sugar; when the crystal sugar is dissolved, turn off the stove, put it aside and let it cool. ❸Add milk and vinegar to egg white and stir gently; pour it into a small bowl, cover it with cling film and put it into a steamer; steam it for about 30 minutes so it turns into cheese; sprinkle the cheese with smashed papaya before serving it.

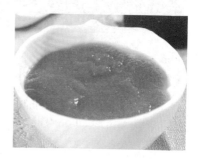

Tangerine

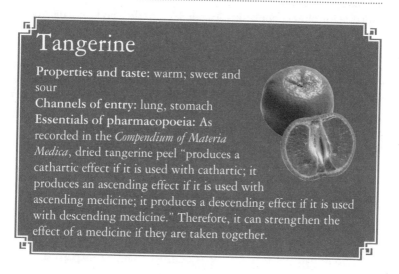

Properties and taste: warm; sweet and sour

Channels of entry: lung, stomach

Essentials of pharmacopoeia: As recorded in the *Compendium of Materia Medica*, dried tangerine peel "produces a cathartic effect if it is used with cathartic; it produces an ascending effect if it is used with ascending medicine; it produces a descending effect if it is used with descending medicine." Therefore, it can strengthen the effect of a medicine if they are taken together.

Health Effects

Reducing blood pressure: The hesperidin in tangerine peels enhances the tenacity of the blood capillaries, reduces blood pressure and expands the coronary arteries, so it effectively helps prevent coronary heart disease and arteriosclerosis.

Protecting and nourishing the skin: Tangerines are rich in vitamin C and citric acid; the former improves complexion while the latter eliminates fatigue.

Points of Attention for Different People

Suitable for beauty pursuers: Tangerines are rich in vitamin C and citric acid, and their functions include improving complexion and eliminating fatigue.

Suitable for patients with hypertension: The tangerine's hesperidin enhances the tenacity of the blood capillaries, reduces blood pressure and expands the coronary arteries.

Suitable for cancer patients: Fresh tangerine juice contains a substance with strong antitumor properties, as it decomposes cancerogenic substances, and inhibits and blocks the growth of cancer cells.

Not suitable for those with excessive internal heat: The tangerine is high in calories; it causes periodontitis if people eat too much of it and get excess internal fire.

Food Compatibility and Incompatibility

Suitable: tangerines + walnuts = helps people to obtain a ruddy complexion and enhances physical strength

Suitable: tangerines + oranges = enhances immunity and prevents colds

Avoid: tangerines + white turnips = inhibits the absorption of iodine

Avoid: tangerines + milk = reduces nutritive value

Eating Tip

Three tangerines satisfies the human body's daily vitamin C requirement. When eating tangerines, many people throw away tangerine pith (fibers on the inside of the peel); but tangerine pith is edible and its functions include promoting the secretion of body fluids, quenching thirst, eliminating phlegm and relieving coughs.

Healthy Recipes
Ginger, Date and Tangerine Juice
Ingredients: 200 g (7 oz)
tangerines, 50 g (2 oz) red dates,
10 g (0.4 oz) ginger, 100 g (3.5 oz)
dringking water

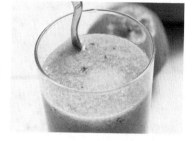

   Preparation: ❶Peel the
tangerines, remove their seeds and
dice them; wash, halve and core the
red dates; wash and shred the ginger. ❷Put the above ingredients into the
juicer, add warm drinking water and start the machine.

Kiwi and Tangerine Juice
Ingredients: 150 g (5 oz) each
kiwis and tangerines, 2 g (0.1 oz)
honey (optional), 100g (3.5 oz)
dringking water

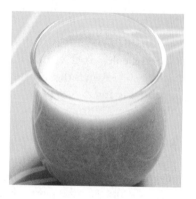

   Preparation: ❶Peel and dice
kiwis and tangerines. ❷Put the
above ingredients into a juicer
and add drinking water; start the
machine, and after it is finished,
season it with some honey.

Watermelon

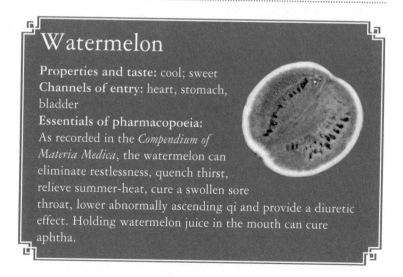

Properties and taste: cool; sweet
Channels of entry: heart, stomach,
bladder
Essentials of pharmacopoeia:
As recorded in the *Compendium of
Materia Medica*, the watermelon can
eliminate restlessness, quench thirst,
relieve summer-heat, cure a swollen sore
throat, lower abnormally ascending qi and provide a diuretic
effect. Holding watermelon juice in the mouth can cure
aphtha.

Health Effects

Relieving restlessness and summer-heat: Watermelon is sweet and juicy. When people have symptoms such as fever, thirst, sweating and restlessness due to acute fever, eating a piece of sweet and juicy watermelon can relieve their symptoms.

Curing nephritis: The sugar and potassium in watermelon provides a diuretic effect, and it relieves symptoms of nephritis; protease transforms insoluble protein into soluble protein and supplements nutrition for the patient with nephritis.

Diminishing inflammation: "Watermelon frost" is made from watermelon peel and can be used to treat aphtha, aphthae, ulcerative gingivitis, acute laryngopharyngitis and other throat diseases.

Protecting the skin: Fresh and tender melon rind helps increase skin elasticity, reduce wrinkles and brighten the complexion.

Points of Attention for Different People

Suitable for beauty pursuers: Fresh watermelon juice and tender melon rind helps increase skin elasticity and smooth wrinkles.

Suitable for patients with hypertension: Watermelon produces a significant antihypertensive effect.

Not suitable for patients with diabetes: Watermelon is high in sugar content.

Food Compatibility and Incompatibility

Suitable: watermelon + mung beans = clears internal heat and relieve summer-heat

Suitable: watermelon + carrots = maintains skin health

Avoid: watermelon + fish = reduces nutritive value

Avoid: watermelon + wine = causes nutrition loss

Eating Tip

Do not eat watermelon immediately after getting it out of the refrigerator; instead, let it warm up to room temperature before eating it, or else it will harm the spleen and stomach functions due to its excess coldness.

Healthy Recipes

Ice-Cold Diced Watermelon

Ingredients: 200 g (7 oz) watermelon flesh; 50 g (2 oz) each pineapple flesh, tangerine sections and apple; 20 g (1 oz) lychees; 2 g (0.1 oz)

crystal sugar; 100 g (3.5 oz) water

Preparation: ❶ Remove seeds of and dice watermelon flesh; dice the pineapple flesh; wash, remove pedicle of, core and dice the apple; wash and peel the lychees. ❷Heat the water and crystal sugar in a pot; when the crystal sugar melts, put it aside;

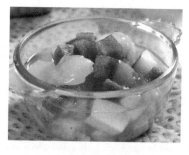

when it cools, store it in the refrigerator for 40 minutes. ❸Put diced watermelon, diced pineapple, split tangerine, diced apple and lychees into a dish and pour the crystal sugar water into the dish.

Watermelon and Strawberry Juice

Ingredients: 150 g (5 oz) watermelon flesh, 100 g (3.5 oz) each strawberries and drinking water

Preparation: ❶ Remove seeds of watermelon and dice it; remove strawberry stems, then wash and dice the straw berries.

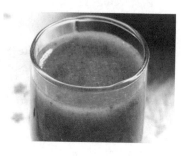

❷Put the ingredients into a juicer and add drinking water for whipping.

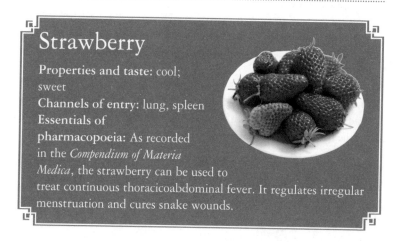

Strawberry

Properties and taste: cool; sweet
Channels of entry: lung, spleen
Essentials of pharmacopoeia: As recorded in the *Compendium of Materia Medica*, the strawberry can be used to treat continuous thoracicoabdominal fever. It regulates irregular menstruation and cures snake wounds.

Health Effects

Clearing away the lung-heat and removing phlegm: The functions of strawberry include moistening the lungs and removing phlegm.

Promoting digestion: Strawberries contain a variety of organic acids and pectic substances, which help indigestion and promote gastrointestinal peristalsis, and its functions also include expelling toxins.

Preventing and fighting cancer: The strawberry is rich in tannic acid, which blocks the absorption of cancerogenic substances by the human body; vitamin C suppresses the generation of nitrosamines, a strong cancerogenic substance, and reduces the morbidity of cancer.

Improving the complexion: Frequent strawberry consumption produces good effects on the skin and hair.

Points of Attention for Different People

Suitable for drunken people: Eating strawberries after drinking wine accelerates the decomposition of ethyl alcohol in the human body.

Not suitable for patients with lithiasis: The strawberry is rich in calcium oxalate, and excessive intake of it will worsen the condition.

Food Compatibility and Incompatibility

Suitable: strawberries + yogurt = supplements nutrition, nourishes the heart and soothes the nerves

Suitable: strawberries + hazelnut = prevents anemia and enhances physical strength

Avoid: strawberries + oats = reduces nutritive value

Avoid: strawberries + sweet potatoes = induces gastrointestinal discomfort

Eating Tip

Before washing strawberries, soak them in saline for about five minutes to maximally kill microorganisms such as bacteria. However, do not soak them too long, or else the pesticides will penetrate the flesh; these have detrimental effects on the body. When washing strawberries, wash them with flowing water, and do not remove the stems, or they will lose vitamin C and their flavor will be reduced.

Healthy Recipes
Strawberry, Grapefruit and Orange Juice

Ingredients: 150 g (5 oz) grapefruit, 50 g (2 oz) each strawberries and oranges; 2 g (0.1 oz) honey; 100 g (3.5 oz) drinking water

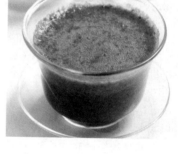

Preparation: ❶Remove stems of and wash the strawberries, and dice them; peel grapefruit and oranges, and dice them. ❷Put the above ingredients into a juicer, add drinking water for whipping, and then add the honey. Dish up after mixing it evenly.

Spinach, Strawberry and Grape Juice

Ingredients: 50 g (2 oz) strawberries, 100 g (3.5 oz) each spinach and grapes, 2 g (0.1 oz) honey, 100 g (3.5 oz) drinking water

Preparation: ❶Wash the spinach, remove its roots and scald it in boiling water; remove, cool, and cut it into strips; wash the grapes and remove their seeds, wash and shred them. ❷Put the above ingredients into a juicer and add drinking water for whipping.

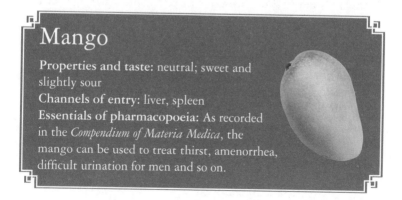

Mango

Properties and taste: neutral; sweet and slightly sour

Channels of entry: liver, spleen

Essentials of pharmacopoeia: As recorded in the *Compendium of Materia Medica*, the mango can be used to treat thirst, amenorrhea, difficult urination for men and so on.

Health Effects

Antimicrobial effects and treating inflammation: Mangoes inhibit pyogenic coccus and E. coli, and they can be used to treat infectious diseases of the skin and digestive tract.

Preventing and fighting cancer: Mangoes contain mangiferonic acid, isomangiferolic acid and polyphenols, and they produce an anticancer effect; mango juice also promotes gastrointestinal peristalsis and effectively prevents and cures colorectal cancer.

Improving eyesight and nourishing the skin: Mangoes are rich in carotene, which is not only good for vision, but also nourishes the skin.

Points of Attention for Different People

Suitable for patients with cardiovascular disease: Frequent mango consumption supplements vitamin C and prevents and cures cardiovascular disease.

Suitable for people with cough and asthma: The mango's functions include eliminating phlegm and relieving a cough.

Not suitable for people of allergic physique: Clean the mango juice from around the lips after eating the mango in case it causes an allergic reaction.

Not suitable for patients with diabetes: Mangoes have a high sugar content.

Food Compatibility and Incompatibility

Suitable: mangoes + milk = protects eyes and prevents cancer
Suitable: mangoes + cheese = promotes calcium absorption
Avoid: mangoes + pork liver = destroys vitamin C
Avoid: mangoes + carrots = destroys vitamin C

Eating Tip

Before eating a mango, peel and dice it; rinse the mouth and wash the face after eating it to effectively prevent mango allergy.

Healthy Recipes
Mango Porridge

Ingredients: 50 g (2 oz) each black rice and rice, 25 g (1 oz) each mango and yogurt, 2 g (0.1 oz) white sugar, 100 g (3.5 oz) water

Preparation: ❶Wash rice and black rice and soak them for 30 minutes and two hours,

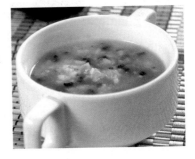

respectively; wash, peel, core and dice the mango for further use.
❷Bring the water to a boil in a pot, then add black rice and rice to the water and boil over high heat. Adjust the heat to low and wait until the rice becomes thoroughly cooked. Add diced mango to the porridge and boil it for five minutes; add some white sugar and stir; dish it up after sprinkling it with yogurt.

Mango, Honey and Milk Drink

Ingredients: 200 g (7 oz) mangos, 300 ml (10 oz) skim milk, 2 g (0.1 oz) honey

Preparation: ❶Peel and core the mangos and dice the flesh. ❷Put the mango and milk into a juicer, start the machine; when it is finished, dish it up and enrich the flavor by adding some honey to it.

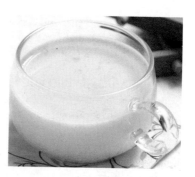

Hawthorn Berry

Properties and taste: slightly warm; sweet and sour
Channels of entry: spleen, stomach, liver
Essentials of pharmacopoeia: As recorded in the *Compendium of Materia Medica*, hawthorn berries eliminate dyspepsia, nourish the spleen, cure hernia of the small intestine and children's shingles, strengthen the stomach and disperse the stagnation of qi.

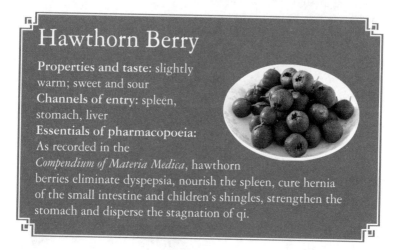

Health Effects

Strengthening the stomach and helping digestion: Hawthorn berries remove food retention and eliminate stagnation, and they contain lipolytic enzymes that promote gastric secretions, increase digestive enzymes inside the stomach, promote the digestion of high-fat foods and reduce the accumulation of cholesterol in the human body.

Activating the blood and dissolving stasis: Hawthorn berries help clear local blood stasis, and they produce an auxiliary effect on traumatic injury; they expedite child delivery for a pregnant woman who eats hawthorn berries when she is about to give birth, and they also promote postpartum uterine involution.

Points of Attention for Different People

Suitable for patients with hypertension: Hawthorn berries can be used to prevent and cure cardiovascular disease, and their functions include reducing blood pressure and cholesterol.

Suitable for people with traumatic injury: The hawthorn berry's functions include activating blood and dissolving stasis.

Not suitable for pregnant women: Hawthorn berries stimulate uterine contractions and they might induce spontaneous abortion.

Not suitable for children: The tartaric acid in hawthorn berries may corrode the teeth.

Food Compatibility and Incompatibility

Suitable: hawthorn berries + malt = helps digestion

Suitable: hawthorn berries + lotus leaves = relieves summer-heat, induces resuscitation and reduces blood pressure

Avoid: hawthorn berries + seafood = causes dyspepsia

Avoid: hawthorn berries + pork liver = affects nutrient absorption

Eating Tip

Gastric concretion will be formed if the tannic acid in fresh hawthorn berries is brought into contact with gastric acid, and it is suggested that the people with weak gastrointestinal functions cook hawthorn berries before eating them.

Healthy Recipes

Hawthorn and Cucumber Juice

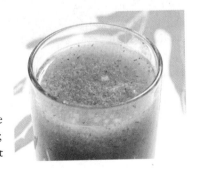

Ingredients: 100 g (3.5 oz) hawthorn berries, 200 g (7 oz) cucumber, 2 g (0.1 oz) honey, 100 g (3.5 oz) drinking water

Preparation: ❶Wash, remove seeds of and dice hawthorn berries; wash and dice the cucumber. ❷Put the hawthorn berries and cucumber into a juicer, add drinking water; start the machine, and when it is finished, add some honey and mix it up evenly.

Hawthorn and Red Date Juice

Ingredients: 100 g (3.5 oz) each hawthorn berries, red dates and drinking water; 2 g (0.1 oz) crystal sugar

Preparation: ❶Wash, core and shred the hawthorn berries and red dates. ❷Add water, hawthorn berries and red dates to the juicer. Start the machine and pour the juice into a glass after the machine stops; add some crystal sugar and dish it up.

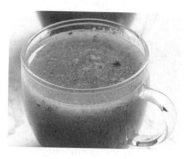

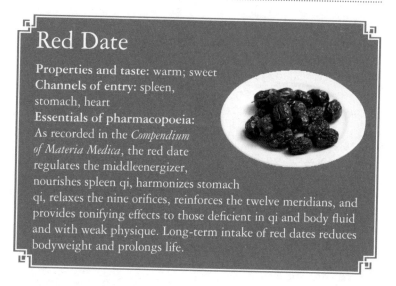

Red Date

Properties and taste: warm; sweet
Channels of entry: spleen, stomach, heart
Essentials of pharmacopoeia: As recorded in the *Compendium of Materia Medica*, the red date regulates the middleenergizer, nourishes spleen qi, harmonizes stomach qi, relaxes the nine orifices, reinforces the twelve meridians, and provides tonifying effects to those deficient in qi and body fluid and with weak physique. Long-term intake of red dates reduces bodyweight and prolongs life.

Health Effects

Strengthening physical fitness: Red dates can be used as an ingredient in cooking all kinds of food, and they produce a tonifying effect, nourish blood, tonify the spleen, benefit qi and improve the body's immunity.

Protecting the liver: The red date contains fructose, glucose, oligosaccharide and acidic polysaccharose, and all these can protect the liver and reduce the damage chemicals cause to the liver.

Preventing anemia: Red dates are rich in calcium and iron, and they provide dietary therapy to the patient with anemia and osteoporosis. Red dates produce a good nourishing effect on patients who are weak and recovering from illness.

Points of Attention for Different People

Suitable for people with anemia and osteoporosis: Red dates are rich in calcium and iron, and they provide good curative effects to people with osteoporosis and anemia.

Suitable for patients with hypertension: Red dates contain rutin, which softens blood vessel and reduces blood pressure.

Not suitable for patients with diabetes: Red dates are high in sugar, so these people should not eat too many red dates.

Not suitable for patients with edema: Eating too much red date produces dampness, and the dampness will accumulate in the human body, worsening edema.

Food Compatibility and Incompatibility

Suitable: red dates + celery = moisturizes the skin and produces an anti-aging effect

Suitable: red dates + tomatoes = restores health and strengthens the stomach

Avoid: red dates + garlic = causes dyspepsia

Cooking Tip

To cook red dates, try to cut single one into three to five pieces if they are to be decocted or stewed, as this helps release their effective components.

Healthy Recipes

Red Dates and Peanut Skin Soup

Ingredients: 50 g (2 oz) red dates, 100 g (3.5 oz) peanuts, 3 g (0.1 oz) brown sugar, 500 g (18 oz) water

Preparation: ❶Wash red dates, soak them in warm water and core them; boil the peanuts for a few minutes, then soak them in

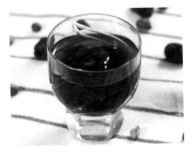

cold water and remove their skins. ❷Put red dates and peanut skins into the pot and add some water to it; when it boils over high heat, adjust the heat to low and boil for 30 minutes; remove the peanut skins, add brown sugar until the soup becomes thick; dish it up.

Pearl Barley, Lotus Seeds and Red Dates Porridge

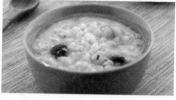

Ingredients: 50 g (2 oz) each pearl barley and rice, 5 g (0.2 oz) each grams of dried lotus seed and dried red dates 500g (18 oz) water

Preparation: ❶Soak pearl barley and dried lotus seeds for about an hour respectively; wash them and put them into the pot. ❷Wash rice and red dates and put them into the pot; add 500 g water; when it boils over high heat, adjust the heat to low and continue to boil; dish it up when the porridge becomes thick and pearl barley is well-cooked.

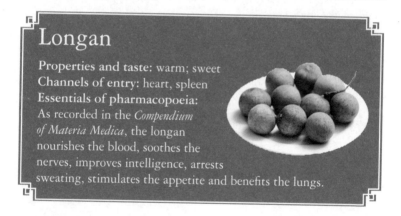

Longan

Properties and taste: warm; sweet
Channels of entry: heart, spleen
Essentials of pharmacopoeia:
As recorded in the *Compendium of Materia Medica*, the longan nourishes the blood, soothes the nerves, improves intelligence, arrests sweating, stimulates the appetite and benefits the lungs.

Health Effects

Tonifying the body: Longans are rich in glucose, saccharose and protein, and they're also high in iron, so besides enhancing heat energy and providing extra nutrition, they promote regeneration of hemoglobin to enrich the blood, and can be used to treat diseases such as palpitations, nervousness, insomnia and amnesia and so on.

Preventing miscarriage and nourishing the fetus: Longans improve the memory and eliminate fatigue, and they are rich in iron elements and vitamin B_2, which help prevent miscarriage.

Preventing cancer: The inhibiting rate of longans against the metrocarcinoma cells exceeds 90 percent, and frequent consumption helps prevent and treat cancer.

Points of Attention for Different People

Suitable for elderly people: Longans produce an anti-aging effect.

Suitable for climacteric women: The inhibiting rate of longan against the metrocarcinoma cells exceeds 90 percent, and longan consumption is good for health.

Suitable for people with insomnia and anemia: Longans are rich in a variety of nutrients, and their functions include enriching the blood, soothing the nerves, and nourishing the heart and spleen.

Not suitable for people with excessive internal heat and inflammation: Longans belong to warm and hot food, and excessive intake may cause stagnation of qi.

Food Compatibility and Incompatibility

Suitable: longans + red dates = enriches and nourishes the blood

Suitable: longans + eggs = soothes the nerves and improves the complexion

Suitable: longans + ginseng = enhances physical strength

Suitable: longans + yams = tonifies the spleen and benefits qi

Eating Tip

Some people eat longans directly after buying them, as they believe that the flesh is clean and there is no need to wash the fruit. Actually, there is dust and bacteria in the peel, which will stick to the flesh when peeling the longan, so wash it thoroughly under flowing water before eating.

Healthy Recipes

Longan and Ginger Porridge

Ingredients: 75 g (3 oz) rice, 40 g (2 oz) black beans, 25 g (1 oz) longans, 20 g (1 oz) fresh ginger, 4 g (0.1 oz) salt, 500 g (18 oz) water

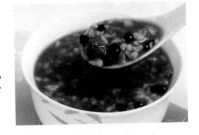

Preparation: ❶Wash rice, longan and black beans and soak black beans for four hours; peel the fresh ginger and grind it. ❷Heat water in a pot, add the black beans to the water and bring to a boil; when it boils, adjust the heat to low and continue to boil for about 20 minutes. Add longan, rice and ginger juice and stir the porridge until it is mixed thoroughly; season it with some salt and dish it up.

Longan and Glutinous Rice Porridge

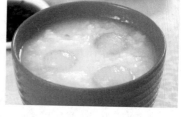

Ingredients: 100 g (3.5 oz) glutinous rice, 15 g (0.5 oz) longan flesh, 2 g (0.1 oz) crystal sugar, 500 g (18 oz) water

Preparation: ❶Wash the glutinous rice and soak it for two hours. ❷Put the glutinous rice in a pot of water and bring it to a boil over high heat. When it boils, reduce the heat to low and continue to boil until the porridge is half-cooked. ❸Add the longan flesh and crystal sugar; stir the porridge until it is thoroughly mixed; when it is well-cooked, dish it up.

Peanut

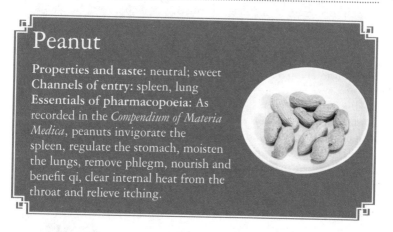

Properties and taste: neutral; sweet
Channels of entry: spleen, lung
Essentials of pharmacopoeia: As recorded in the *Compendium of Materia Medica*, peanuts invigorate the spleen, regulate the stomach, moisten the lungs, remove phlegm, nourish and benefit qi, clear internal heat from the throat and relieve itching.

Health Effects

Reducing cholesterol: Peanuts contain unsaturated fatty acid, which decomposes the cholesterol in the human body into bile acid and allows it to be excreted from the body to prevent coronary heart disease and arteriosclerosis.

Hemostasis: Peanuts and their peels are rich in vitamin K, which provides a hemostasis function, and it also produces a good curative effect on a variety of hemorrhagic disease and anemia caused by hemorrhage.

Invigorating the brain and moisturizing the skin: Peanuts contain vitamin E and zinc, and they improve the memory, produce an anti-aging effect, postpone senescence of the brain functions and moisturize the skin.

Points of Attention for Different People

Suitable for patients with cardiovascular disease: The unsaturated fatty acid in peanuts reduces cholesterol and helps prevent diseases such as hypertension, coronary heart disease and atherosclerosis.

Suitable for children: Peanuts are rich in calcium, which promotes bone health.

Suitable for parturients: Peanuts nourishes qi and blood and promote lactation.

Not suitable for obese people: Peanuts are high in fat, and it is not suggested that obese people eat too much of them.

Food Compatibility and Incompatibility

Suitable: peanuts + shrimp = strengthens the bones and teeth

Suitable: peanuts + fish = strengthens calcium absorption

Avoid: peanuts + beef tallow = causes dyspepsia

Avoid: Peanuts + crabs = causes diarrhea

Cooking Tip

It is suggested that the peanuts be stewed, because stewing makes them tender, soft, tasty and digestible, and it prevents their nutrients from being lost or destroyed in the cooking process.

Healthy Recipes

Peanuts Porridge

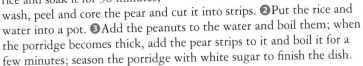

Ingredients: 100 g (3.5 oz) rice, 30 g (1 oz) peanuts, one pear, 2 g (0.1 oz) white sugar, 500 g (18 oz) water

Preparation: ❶ Wash the rice and soak it for 30 minutes; wash, peel and core the pear and cut it into strips. ❷Put the rice and water into a pot. ❸Add the peanuts to the water and boil them; when the porridge becomes thick, add the pear strips to it and boil it for a few minutes; season the porridge with white sugar to finish the dish.

Lotus Seed, Peanut and Soy Milk

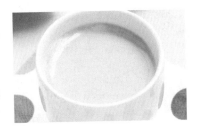

Ingredients: 50 g (2 oz) soybeans, 25 g (1 oz) lotus seeds, 20 g (0.1 oz) peanuts, 10 g (0.4 oz) crystal sugar

Preparation: ❶ Soak soybeans in clean water for eight to twelve hours, then wash them; wash lotus seeds and peanuts and soak them for two hours. ❷Put the above ingredients into the automatic soy milk maker, and feed water into it until it reaches between the upper and lower water lines; press the "soybean milk" button; when the soy milk maker indicates that it is done, strain the soy milk, and stir the crystal sugar into it until it is dissolved.

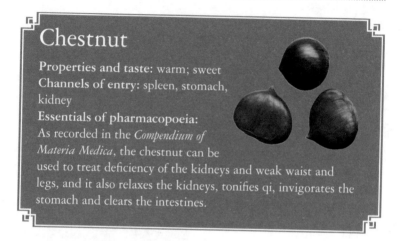

Chestnut

Properties and taste: warm; sweet
Channels of entry: spleen, stomach, kidney
Essentials of pharmacopoeia:
As recorded in the *Compendium of Materia Medica*, the chestnut can be used to treat deficiency of the kidneys and weak waist and legs, and it also relaxes the kidneys, tonifies qi, invigorates the stomach and clears the intestines.

Health Effects

Ideal tonic: The restorative functions of the chestnut match that of ginseng, astragalus membranaceus and angelica sinensis. It is rich in unsaturated fatty acid, vitamins and inorganic salt, which provide anti-aging effects and prolong life.

Tonifying the kidney: Eating one or two fresh chestnuts in the morning and at night treats diseases such as soreness and weakness of waist and knees, paralyzed waist and limbs, frequent urination and fracture and pain caused by kidney deficiency.

Strengthening the spleen and stomach functions: Chestnuts are rich in carbohydrates, and they produce an energizing effect on the human body and promote fat metabolism. The chestnut's functions include tonifying qi, tonifying spleen, and thickening and nourishing the stomach and intestines.

Points of Attention for Different People

Suitable for elderly people: Chestnuts provide anti-aging effects and prolong life.

Suitable for patients with dental ulcers: The vitamin B_2 in chestnuts is beneficial to the treatment of dental ulcers.

Not suitable for people with dyspepsia: Chestnuts are indigestible, and they may cause stagnation of qi.

Not suitable for patients with diabetes: Chestnuts are high in sugar content.

Food Compatibility and Incompatibility

Suitable: chestnuts + corn = helps digestion

Suitable: chestnuts + grapefruit = protects against the cold and promotes wound healing

Suitable: chestnuts + chicken = nourishes the spleen and produces a hematopoiesis effect.

Avoid: chestnuts + beef = reduces nutritional value

Eating Tip

Chestnuts are indigestible, and it is suggested that people eat only five chestnuts a day, as more can cause abdominal distension. Besides, the chestnut is rich in starch and eating too much of it after meals will result in the intake of excessive calories, so those on a diet should pay special attention how mang chestnuts they consume.

Healthy Recipes

Sesame and Chestnut Paste

Ingredients: 100 g (3.5 oz) cooked chestnuts, 50 g (2 oz) cooked black sesame

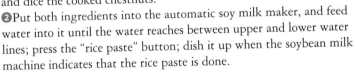

Preparation: ❶Shell, peel and dice the cooked chestnuts. ❷Put both ingredients into the automatic soy milk maker, and feed water into it until the water reaches between upper and lower water lines; press the "rice paste" button; dish it up when the soybean milk machine indicates that the rice paste is done.

Chestnut, Oat and Soybean Milk

Ingredients: 60 g (2 oz) soybeans, 50 g (2 oz) cooked chestnuts, 20 g (1 oz) oatmeal, 15 g (0.5 oz) crystal sugar (optional)

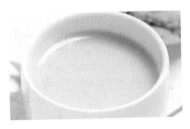

Preparation: ❶Soak soybeans in clean water for eight

to twelve hours and then wash them; shell, peel and dice the cooked chestnuts. ❷Put all ingredients into the automatic soy milk maker, and feed water into it until the water reaches between the upper and lower water lines. Press the "soybean milk" button; when the soy milk maker indicates that the soy milk is done, sieve it and pour it into a glass, then stir crystal sugar into it until it is dissolved.

Walnut

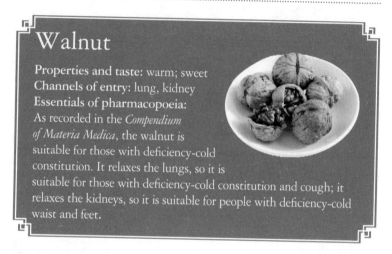

Properties and taste: warm; sweet
Channels of entry: lung, kidney
Essentials of pharmacopoeia:
As recorded in the *Compendium of Materia Medica*, the walnut is suitable for those with deficiency-cold constitution. It relaxes the lungs, so it is suitable for those with deficiency-cold constitution and cough; it relaxes the kidneys, so it is suitable for people with deficiency-cold waist and feet.

Health Effects

Invigorating the brain and improving intelligence: Walnuts are rich in protein and unsaturated fatty acid, which are essential elements of human body; these components nourish brain cells and enhance brain functions.

Preventing and curing senile diseases: Walnuts contain arginine, oleic acid and antioxidants, which are helpful in protecting against angiocarpy, coronary heart disease, stroke and senile dementia.

Moisturizing the skin and protecting the hair: Walnuts are rich in vitamin E, which moisturizes and smooths the skin, making skin more elastic.

Points of Attention for Different People

Suitable for beauty pursuers: Walnuts nourish and brighten the skin.

Suitable for elderly people: Walnuts contain vitamin E, which is a well-known anti-aging substance.

Suitable for knowledge workers: The phospholipids and proteins in walnuts produce a health-care effect and improve the memory.

Not suitable for people with excessive internal heat and diarrhea: Walnuts are high in grease, and too much consumption will cause excessive internal heat and nausea.

Food Compatibility and Incompatibility
Suitable: walnuts + lily bulbs = moistens the lungs, invigorates the kidneys, relieves a cough and relieves asthma

Suitable: walnuts + hawthorn berries = prevents arteriosclerosis

Avoid: walnuts + spirits = produces phlegm and induces restlessness

Avoid: walnuts + bean curd = causes abdominal distension and stomachache

Cooking Tip
Do not peel the light-yellow skin of walnut, or else some nutrients will be lost. Although the fat walnut contains is unsaturated fatty acid, which helps clear away cholesterol, the walnut is high in calories; excessive consumption of it will result in fat accumulation if it isn't well-utilized. It is suggested that people eat four or five walnuts a day.

Healthy Recipes
Peanut, Walnut and Milk Paste

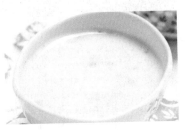

Ingredients: 50 g (2 oz) rice flour, 5 g (0.2 oz) peanuts, 20 g (1 oz) walnuts, 250 ml (9 oz) milk

Preparation: ❶Wash peanuts and walnuts. ❷Mix the milk and rice flour, and pour the mixed rice flour, peanuts and walnuts into the automatic soy milk maker. ❸Feed some water into the machine until the water reaches between upper and lower water lines; press the button for "rice paste," and it is ready when the automatic soy milk maker indicates that the rice paste is done.

Walnut, Sesame and Soybean Milk

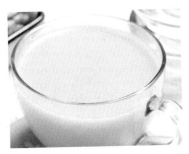

Ingredients: 55 g (2 oz) soybeans, 10 g (0.4 oz) walnuts, 5 g (0.2 oz) cooked black sesame, 10 g (0.4 oz) crystal sugar (optional)

Preparation: ❶Soak the soy for eight to twelve hours and then wash it; pulverize the black sesame; dice the walnuts. ❷Put soybeans, black sesame shreds and walnuts into the automatic soy milk maker, and feed water into it until the water reaches between upper and lower water lines. ❸Press the "soybean milk" button; when the soy milk maker indicates that the soy milk is done, sieve the soy milk, and stir crystal sugar into it until it is dissolved.

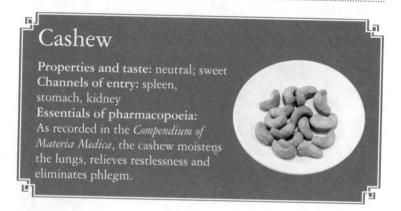

Cashew

Properties and taste: neutral; sweet
Channels of entry: spleen, stomach, kidney
Essentials of pharmacopoeia:
As recorded in the *Compendium of Materia Medica*, the cashew moistens the lungs, relieves restlessness and eliminates phlegm.

Health Effects

Expelling toxins and nourishing the skin: Cashews are rich in grease, with functions including lubricating the intestines, relaxing the bowels, expelling toxins, nourishing the skin and delaying senescence; they also help arouse sexual desire and maintain youth. Frequent cashew consumption effectively prevents and cures cardiovascular and cerebrovascular diseases.

Replenishing energy: Elderly people with inadequate vitamin intake and elderly people who rarely eat meat should eat cashews frequently. It is suggested that people eat three to five cashew a day, and add some cashews to the daily diet to supplement energy and unsaturated fatty acid.

Points of Attention for Different People

Suitable for beauty pursuers: Cashews are rich in grease, and they have skin moisturizing and complexion improving effects, and delay senescence.

Suitable for manual workers: Cashews are rich in vitamin B_1, and their functions include replenishing energy and eliminating fatigue.

Suitable for women with hypogalactia: The cashew's functions include promotion of lactation, and consumption is beneficial to women with low milk production after delivery.

Not suitable for obese people: Cashews are high in grease and can cause obesity if people eat too much.

Food Compatibility and Incompatibility
Suitable: cashews + shrimp = nourishes the hair and relieves arthritis

Suitable: cashews + garlic = nourishes the skin and eliminates fatigue

Avoid: cashews + wine = tends to cause fatty liver

Avoid: cashews + clams = destroys vitamin B_1

Eating Tip
Although the fat in cashews is a benign fatty acid, they are still a high-lipid food, high in calories. Therefore, it is suggested that people not eat more than 15 cashews a day.

Healthy Recipes
Cashew and Peanut Paste
Ingredients: 50 g (2 oz) rice, 25 g (1 oz) cashews, 20 g (1 oz) peanuts

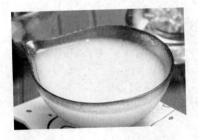

Preparation: ❶Wash the rice and soak it for two hours. ❷Put rice, cashews and peanuts into the automatic soy milk maker, and feed water into the machine until the water reaches between the upper and the lower water lines; press the "rice paste" button; pour it into a glass when the soy milk maker indicates that the rice paste is done.

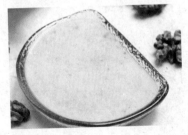

Walnut, Cashew and Rice Paste
Ingredients: 30 g (1 oz) each rice and millet, 10 g (0.4 oz) walnuts, 20 g (1 oz) cashews, 5 g (0.2 oz) each red dates and longans, 10 g (0.4 oz) crystal sugar (optional)

Preparation: ❶Wash rice and millet and soak them for two hours; shred walnuts and cashews; wash and core the red dates; peel and core the longans. ❷Put the above ingredients into the automatic soy milk maker, and feed water into the machine until the water reaches between the upper and lower water lines; press the "rice paste" button; when the soy milk maker indicates that the rice paste is done, stir some crystal sugar into the paste until it is dissolved.

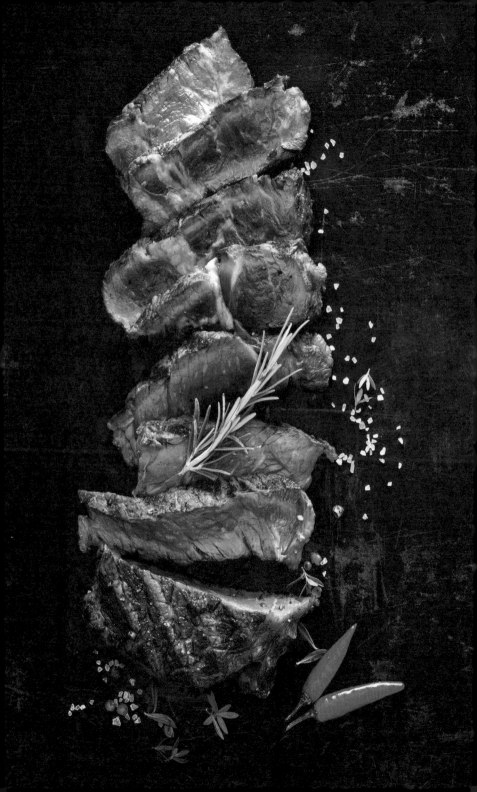

Chapter Five

Meat and Eggs

Meat and eggs replenish energy, help build the body and promote growth and development, and they taste more delicious and mellow than vegetables and fruits. Meanwhile, they are high in fat and rich in protein and essential amino acids. When paired with vegetables in well-balanced meals, meat and eggs are part of a healthy diet.

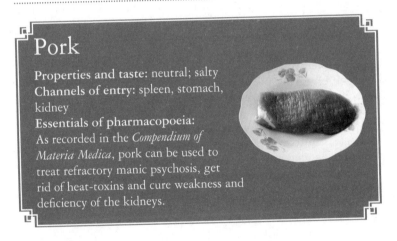

Pork

Properties and taste: neutral; salty
Channels of entry: spleen, stomach, kidney
Essentials of pharmacopoeia:
As recorded in the *Compendium of Materia Medica*, pork can be used to treat refractory manic psychosis, get rid of heat-toxins and cure weakness and deficiency of the kidneys.

Health Effects

Bodybuilding: Pork contains complete protein, which satisfies the body's needs during growth and development; in particular, lean pork protein provides essential amino acids that are not found in bean protein, while pork fat provides calories.

Enriching the blood and nourishing the blood: Pork provides heme iron (organic iron) and cysteine, which promote the body's absorption of iron, and all these substances effectively improve iron-deficiency anemia.

Points of Attention for Different People

Suitable for women: Pigskin and pig trotter are rich in collagen and elastin, which moisturize the skin.

Suitable for people with anemia: Pork provides iron elements and cysteine that promote the absorption of iron, so it helps prevent and cure iron-deficiency anemia.

Food Compatibility and Incompatibility

Suitable: pork + chilis = eliminates fatigue and pain

Suitable: pork + Chinese cabbage = provides extra nutrition and helps digestion

Suitable: pork + turnips = enhances physical strength and promotes defecation

Avoid: pork + tea = tends to cause constipation

Cooking Tip

Stewing pork for an extended time can lower its fat 30 to 50 percent and increase its unsaturated fatty acid, as well as lower its cholesterol content greatly, so a long stewing time is suggested for pork.

Healthy Recipes

Taro and Lean Meat Porridge

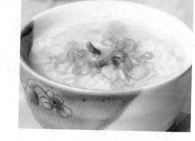

Ingredients: 50 g (2 oz) each rice, taro and lean pork; 2 g (0.1 oz) each chopped scallions, rice wine, salt, sesame oil, monosodium glutamate and black pepper; 500 g (18 oz) boiled water

Preparation: ❶Peel, wash and scald the taro, remove it and dice it; wash and dice the pork; wash the rice, then boil until it becomes porridge. ❷Heat some sesame oil in a pan, then add diced pork and stir-fry. When it is cooked, add some rice wine to it. ❸Add the diced pork and diced taro to the porridge pot and boil; when the porridge becomes thick, season with salt and monosodium glutamate, and sprinkle with chopped scallions.

Braised Pork in Soy Sauce

Ingredients: 500 g (18 oz) pork belly; 2 g (0.1 oz) each chopped green onions, black pepper, anise, dried pimiento strips, white sugar, salt and monosodium glutamate; 20 g (1 oz) vegetable oil

Preparation: ❶Wash and dice the pork, scald it in 300 g (11 oz) boiling water, then remove and wash it. ❷Heat vegetable oil in a pan,

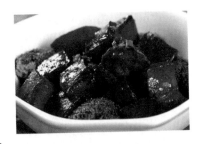

add sugar until it turns brown;
add anise, chopped green onions,
pepper and dried pimiento strips,
and stir-fry them until fragrant.
❸ Put the cooked pork into the
pan and stir-fry it; add white
sugar and 500 g (18 oz) water to
it, and bring to a boil over high
heat; when it boils, adjust the heat
to low, and boil until the pork is well-done; when the soup becomes
thick in the pan, season it with salt and monosodium glutamate.

Beef

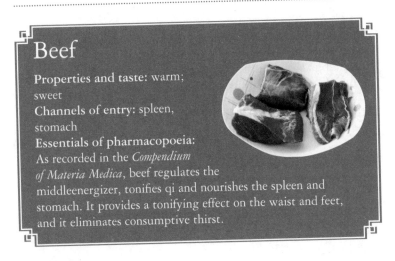

Properties and taste: warm;
sweet
Channels of entry: spleen,
stomach
Essentials of pharmacopoeia:
As recorded in the *Compendium
of Materia Medica*, beef regulates the
middleenergizer, tonifies qi and nourishes the spleen and
stomach. It provides a tonifying effect on the waist and feet,
and it eliminates consumptive thirst.

Health Effects

Building muscle: Beef is rich in sarcosine, which is known as the
"source of muscle energy," and the beef is transformed into energy in
the human body immediately when it is absorbed, enhancing strength
and building muscle.

Restoring deficiency and warming the stomach: Beef is rich in
protein and amino acids, and it improves the body's disease resistance;
as its functions include enriching and nourishing blood and repairing
tissues, it is an ideal food for patients recovering from diseases. When
people eat beef in the winter, it warms the stomach and is an ideal tonic.

Invigorating the brain and improving the intelligence: Beef is
rich in sarcosine, which provides the energy involved in the activities of
brain cells, so it is beneficial to the brain.

Points of Attention for Different People

Suitable for pregnant women and parturients: Beef is rich in iron, which can be easily absorbed by the body, and it effectively prevents the iron-deficient anemia during pregnancy. Beef is quite helpful in treating yin deficiency, nourishing blood and repairing tissues, especially for postpartum women.

Suitable for students: The sarcosine that beef contains improves intelligence.

Not suitable for patients with hyperlipidemia: Beef contains certain amount of cholesterol.

Not suitable for patients with skin disease: Beef is a stimulating food.

Food Compatibility and Incompatibility

Suitable: beef + onions = improves thecomplexion and eliminates fatigue

Suitable: beef + green peppers = prevents arteriosclerosis

Avoid: beef + pork = tends to cause dyspepsia

Avoid: beef + chestnuts = tends to cause gastrointestinal discomfort

Avoid: beef + wine = tends to cause fatty liver

Cooking Tip

Beef shrinks when it is cooked, so cutting it into large chunks prevents it from shrinking into too-small pieces. The muscle fiber of beef is rough, so it is difficult to make it soft and tender; adding some meat tenderizer to it before cooking will improve its texture.

Healthy Recipes

Tomatoes and Beef

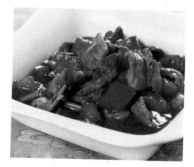

Ingredients: 250 g (9 oz) tomatoes; 50 g (2 oz) lean beef; 2 g (0.1 oz) each chopped green onion, bruised ginger, salt, yellow rice wine, soy sauce, Sichuan pepper powder and monosodium glutamate; 15 g (0.5 oz) vegetable oil

Preparation: ❶Wash the tomatoes, remove their stems and dice them; wash and dice the beef, and mix it with yellow rice wine and soy sauce, and marinate it for 20 minutes. ❷Heat vegetable oil in a pan; when the oil is 70 percent heated, add chopped green onions, bruised ginger and Sichuan pepper powder to it and stir-fry until fragrant. ❸Put diced beef into the pan, stir-fry it and pour some water into the pan; when the beef is 90 percent cooked, add the diced tomato to the pan and boil until it is cooked; dish it up after seasoning it with salt and monosodium glutamate.

Potato and Beef Soup

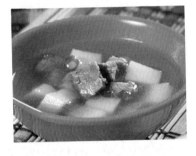

Ingredients: 150 g (5 oz) potatoes; 50 g (2 oz) silverside beef; 2 g (0.1 oz) each minced coriander, chopped green onions, bruised ginger, salt and monosodium glutamate; 15 g (0.5 oz) vegetable oil; 500 g (18 oz) water

Preparation: ❶Peel, wash and dice the potatoes; remove the fascia of silverside, wash and dice it, and scald it in boiling water to remove the bloody water. ❷Heat some vegetable oil in a pan; when the oil is 70 percent heated, add chopped green onions and bruised ginger to the pan and stir-fry until fragrant; add diced beef and fry until it is done. ❸Put the diced potatoes into the pan and stir-fry; pour clean water into the pan, boil until the diced potatoes are well-cooked; season with salt and monosodium glutamate, and sprinkle with minced coriander.

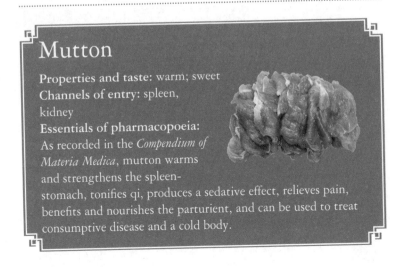

Mutton

Properties and taste: warm; sweet
Channels of entry: spleen, kidney
Essentials of pharmacopoeia:
As recorded in the *Compendium of Materia Medica*, mutton warms and strengthens the spleen-stomach, tonifies qi, produces a sedative effect, relieves pain, benefits and nourishes the parturient, and can be used to treat consumptive disease and a cold body.

Health Effects

Resisting disease and prolonging life: Mutton is tender and digestible, and frequent mutton consumption enhances physical fitness and disease resistance capability.

Ideal tonic in winter: Lamb is a warm tonic that nourishes kidney yang and benefits blood and qi, and its functions include eliminating dampness, warming the heart and stomach, invigorating the kidneys, and tonifying yang.

Points of Attention for Different People

Suitable for elderly people: Frequent mutton consumption relieves the symptoms such as tinnitus and blurred vision, as well as waist-leg weakness.

Suitable for males: The functions of mutton include reinforcing kidney-yang, nourishing essence and blood, invigorating the kidneys and tonifying yang.

Suitable for parturients: Mutton can be used to treat postpartum blood deficiency and stomachache, affection by cold or low milk supply after delivery.

Not suitable for patients with fever: Mutton is warm in properties, so it can worsen the condition.

Food Compatibility and Incompatibility

Suitable: mutton + bean curd = reduces cholesterol and prevents excessive internal heat

Avoid: mutton + tea = causes constipation

Avoid: mutton + vinegar = causes diarrhea

Avoid: mutton + watermelon = causes imbalance of the spleen and stomach functions

Cooking Tip

Mutton gives off a special smell, which can be dissipated if several hawthorn berries, some radishes or mung beans are added when boiling the mutton or seasonings like green onions, ginger and cumin are added when frying the mutton.

Healthy Recipe

Quick-Fried Mutton Slices with Scallions

Ingredients: 200 g (7 oz) mutton hindquarter; two scallions; three garlic cloves; 3 g (0.1 oz) each rice wine, soy sauce, white sugar, white pepper powder, vinegar and salt; 20 g (1 oz) vegetable oil

Preparation: ❶Pluck the green leaves of scallions and keep the white part; wash and cut it into small strips; peel and wash the garlic, then smash it with the back of a knife blade. ❷Wash and slice the mutton, and season it with rice wine, soy sauce, sugar and white pepper powder and marinate it for 10 minutes. ❸Heat some oil in a pan and when the oil is 80 percent heated, add the sliced lamb to the pan; stir-fry it until the color of the lamb changes. After stir-frying it for 15 minutes, add scallion strips to the pan and sprinkle it with a spoonful of vinegar; put garlic and salt into the pan and stir-fry it evenly.

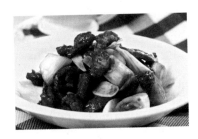

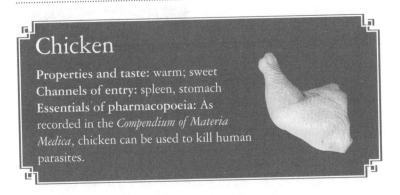

Chicken

Properties and taste: warm; sweet
Channels of entry: spleen, stomach
Essentials of pharmacopoeia: As recorded in the *Compendium of Materia Medica*, chicken can be used to kill human parasites.

Health Effects

Building the body: Chicken is rich in a variety of proteins that are easily absorbed by the body, and also constitutes an important source of fat and phospholipids. The functions of chicken include enhancing physical strength and producing a bodybuilding effect.

Warming the spleen-stomach and tonifying deficiency: Chicken is warm in properties, and it tastes sweet. Its functions include warming the spleen-stomach to tonify qi, restoring deficiency to replenish essence, strengthening the spleen and stomach, and building muscles and bones. In addition, it provides good dietary therapy for symptoms such as malnutrition, intolerance of cold weather, feebleness, fatigue, irregular menstruation, etc.

Enriching the blood and protecting the skin: The chicken breast is rich in B vitamins, which helps eliminate fatigue and protect the skin; the drumsticks are rich in iron, which helps treat iron-deficiency anemia.

Points of Attention for Different People

Suitable for physically weak people: Chicken soothes the nerves, invigorates the five internal organs and enhances physical strength.

Suitable for women: Chicken can be used to treat diseases such as metrorrhagia, metrostaxis, morbid leucorrhea and postpartum agalactia.

Food Compatibility and Incompatibility

Suitable: chicken + green onions = refreshes the mind

Suitable: chicken + green peppers = prevents arteriosclerosis

Suitable: chicken + cabbage = prevents anemia

Suitable: chicken + mushrooms = prevents stroke and colorectal cancer

Avoid: chicken + mustard = tends to cause excessive internal heat and devitalize human body

Healthy Recipes

Steamed Chicken with Mushrooms

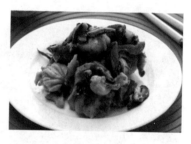

Ingredients: 250 g (9 oz) chicken; 100 g (3.5 oz) water-swollen mushrooms; 20 g (1 oz) each salt, rice wine, monosodium glutamate, soy sauce, sliced scallion, shredded ginger, water starch and clear soup; 4 g (0.1 oz) sesame oil

Preparation: ❶ Wash and slice the chicken; wash and shred the water-swollen mushrooms. ❷ Put chicken and mushrooms into a bowl and season them with soy sauce, salt, monosodium glutamate, sliced scallion, shredded ginger, rice wine, clear soup and water starch, and mix them up; steam it in a steamer and remove when it is cooked; dish it up and sprinkle the dish with sesame oil.

Chicken and Tomato Soup

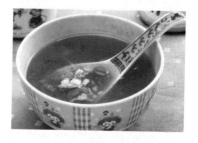

Ingredients: 25 g (1 oz) chicken breast; one tomato; 2 g (0.1 oz) each salt, water starch and sesame oil; 500 g (18 oz) water

Preparation: ❶ Wash and mince the chicken breast; wash, remove stem of, peel and shred the tomato. ❷ Put minced chicken, tomato and water in a pot; bring it to a boil, then adjust the heat to low and boil for 10 minutes; add some salt to it and thicken with mixture of cornstarch and water; sprinkle it with sesame oil.

Duck

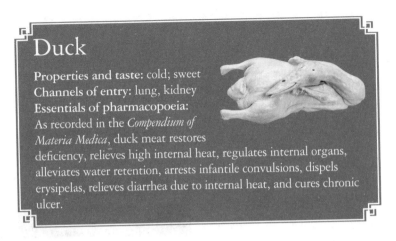

Properties and taste: cold; sweet
Channels of entry: lung, kidney
Essentials of pharmacopoeia:
As recorded in the *Compendium of Materia Medica*, duck meat restores deficiency, relieves high internal heat, regulates internal organs, alleviates water retention, arrests infantile convulsions, dispels erysipelas, relieves diarrhea due to internal heat, and cures chronic ulcer.

Health Effects

Easing swelling, removing phlegm and relieving a cough: The functions of duck meat include curing consumptive disease, clearing away lung-heat to bring down internal heat, relieving a cough and removing phlegm, nourishing the stomach and promoting fluid production, treating yin deficiency and enriching the blood, arresting convulsions, detoxifying the body and eliminating edema.

Protecting blood vessel: Duck meat is rich in unsaturated fatty acid and low-carbon fatty acid, which helps reduce cholesterol and protect the heart and cerebral vessels.

Diminishing inflammation: Duck meat is rich in B vitamins, which help maintain normal functions of human metabolism, nerves, heart, digestion and vision, and also helps the body resist inflammation.

Points of Attention for Different People

Suitable for parturients: Frequent consumption of duck meat helps improve postpartum agalactia.

Suitable for patients with diabetes: Duck meat strengthens the spleen and stomach and tonifies the lungs and kidneys. It is an ideal food for patients with diabetes and lung dryness or stomach heat.

Not suitable for people with weak spleen and stomach functions: Duck meat is cold in properties.

Food Compatibility and Incompatibility

Suitable: duck meat + ginger = warms the body and stimulates blood circulation

Suitable: duck meat + yams = eliminates the oily feel of greasy food, tonifies the spleen and quenches thirst

Avoid: duck meat + walnuts = reduces nutritive value

Cooking Tip
It is difficult to thoroughly cook old duck meat; add some papaya peels to the soup, as an enzyme contained in the papaya can accelerate the cooking of the meat.

Healthy Recipe
Duck Meat with Fermented Glutinous Rice

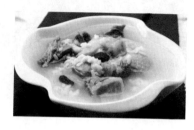

Ingredients: Half of a duck; 150 g (5 oz) fermented glutinous rice; 2 g (0.1 oz) each Chinese wolfberries, white pepper powder, salt and monosodium glutamate

Preparation: ❶ Wash and dice the duck meat, season it with Chinese wolfberries, white pepper powder, salt and monosodium glutamate, pour fermented glutinous rice into the pot; put on disposable gloves and mix all these ingredients, then refrigerate it for four to five hours. ❷ Place the duck meat with fermented glutinous rice in the microwave oven and cook it with high heat for 30 minutes.

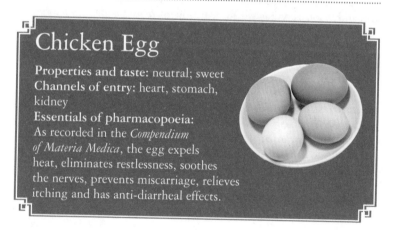

Chicken Egg

Properties and taste: neutral; sweet
Channels of entry: heart, stomach, kidney
Essentials of pharmacopoeia:
As recorded in the *Compendium of Materia Medica*, the egg expels heat, eliminates restlessness, soothes the nerves, prevents miscarriage, relieves itching and has anti-diarrheal effects.

Health Effects
Invigorating the brain and improving intelligence: The egg is rich in DHA and lecithin and it has great effect on the nervous system and physical development, as it invigorates the brain and improves brain health and memory.

Prolonging life: The egg contains almost all the nutrients the body needs. When those longevous persons share their experiences, it has been found that their secret of prolonging life is to eat an egg a day.

Points of Attention for Different People

Not suitable for patients with hepatopathy and gallbladder disorder: The cholesterol and fat in eggs are metabolized in liver, which overloads the liver.

Not suitable for patients with hyperpyrexia: For the patients with hyperpyrexia have decreased secretion of digestive juices, and their digestive abilities are reduced. The egg is high in protein, and it is indigestible, so it can cause dyspepsia symptoms such as abdominal distension and diarrhea, etc., which is not beneficial for the patient's recovery.

Food Compatibility and Incompatibility

Suitable: eggs + tomatoes = bodybuilding and anti-aging

Suitable: eggs + loofahs = brings down a fever, gets rid of toxins, enriches the blood and promotes lactation

Avoid: eggs + tangerines = causes dyspepsia

Avoid: eggs + monosodium glutamate = spoils the deliciousness of the egg

Cooking Tip

It isn't suggested that people eat raw eggs, because the avidin and antitrypsin in raw eggs prevents the human body from breaking down and absorbing the nutrients. Healthy cooking methods include boiling eggs, egg flower soup and steamed eggs.

Healthy Recipe

Yolk Soup

Ingredients: One egg yolk, 2 g (0.1 oz) each salt and sesame oil, 50 ml (2 oz) water

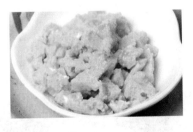

Preparation: ❶Pour yolk into a heat-resistant bowl and whip it; add salt and 50 ml clean water and mix it evenly. ❷Turn on the stove and place the steaming pot on it. Pour some water into the pot and put the steaming curtain on it; place the bowl loaded with yolk and put the cover on the pot; when the water boils, steam it for eight minutes; sprinkle it with sesame oil.

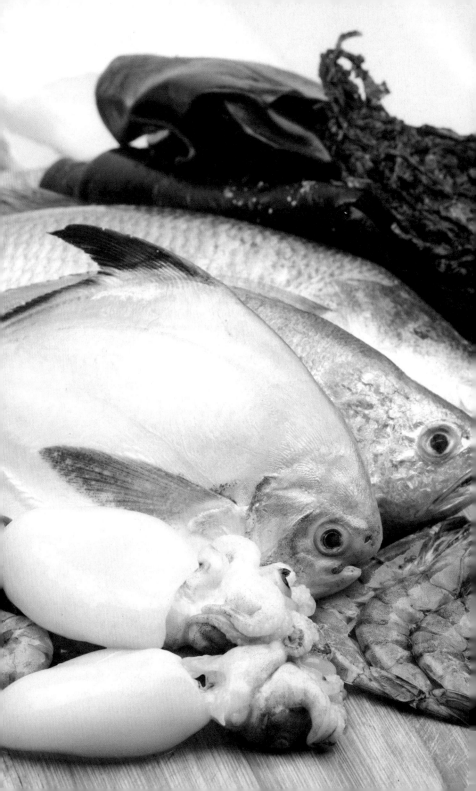

Chapter Six

Aquatic Products

When it comes to aquatic products, we always think of "fresh and delicious." Fish, shrimp and crabs satisfy our appetites, but we need to pay attention to food pairing and preparation in case they cause discomfort to our bodies.

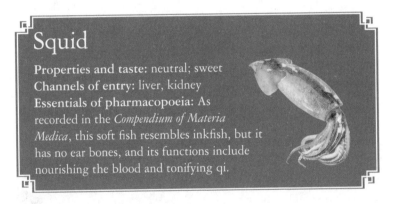

Squid

Properties and taste: neutral; sweet
Channels of entry: liver, kidney
Essentials of pharmacopoeia: As recorded in the *Compendium of Materia Medica*, this soft fish resembles inkfish, but it has no ear bones, and its functions include nourishing the blood and tonifying qi.

Health Effects

Enriching the blood and moisturizing the skin: The squid is rich in protein and nutrients essential to the human body such as amino acids, calcium, phosphorus and iron, etc. Its functions include treating yin deficiency, nourishing the stomach, enriching the blood and moisturizing the skin, and it is quite good for skeletal development and the hemopoietic system.

Delaying senescence: The functions of squid include regulating blood pressure, protecting nerve fibers and activating cells, and frequent intake delays senescence.

Expelling toxins: Other functions of squid include detoxification and expulsion of toxins, and it also improves liver functions.

Radioresistance: Micro-elements in squid such as polypeptides and selenium produce antiviral and antiradiation effects.

Points of Attention for Different People

Suitable for people with anemia: Eating squid promotes hematopoiesis and prevents anemia.

Suitable for patients with hepatopathy: Squid is rich in taurine, and it relieves fatigue and improves liver function.

Not suitable for patients with cardiovascular disease: The squid is high in cholesterol, and it isn't suggested for these people.

Food Compatibility and Incompatibility

Suitable: squid + chilis = balances nutrition and helps digestion

Suitable: squid + corn = improves the efficacy of vitamin B_6

Avoid: squid + tea = reduces the absorption of protein

Avoid: squid + tomatoes = overburdens the kidneys

Cooking Tip

Do not eat squid before it is thoroughly cooked. Because the squid contains polypeptides, eating it when it's undercooked causes peristalsis imbalance.

Healthy Recipe

Spicy Fried Squid Ring

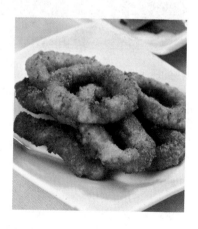

Ingredients: 300 g (11 oz) fresh squid; one egg; 5 g (0.2 oz) breadcrumbs; 30 g (1 oz) vegetable oil; 2 g (0.1 oz) each salt, ground pepper, starch and ketchup

Preparation: ❶Wash the squid and cut it into rings; season it with salt and ground pepper and set it aside for a few minutes. ❷Break and whip the egg; dip the squid rings in a little starch, egg liquid and breadcrumbs successively. ❸Heat some oil in a pan, then add the squid rings and fry until they become crispy and golden; get them out and dish them up, and serve with ketchup.

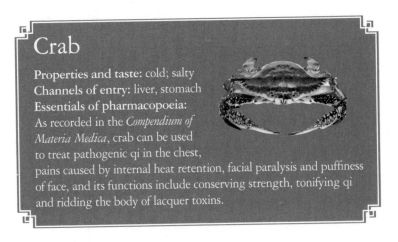

Crab

Properties and taste: cold; salty
Channels of entry: liver, stomach
Essentials of pharmacopoeia:
As recorded in the *Compendium of Materia Medica*, crab can be used to treat pathogenic qi in the chest, pains caused by internal heat retention, facial paralysis and puffiness of face, and its functions include conserving strength, tonifying qi and ridding the body of lacquer toxins.

Health Effects

Nourishing the body: Crab is rich in nutrient contents such as protein and microelements, etc., and it produces good nourishing effects on the human body.

Antituberculous: Crab also has an antituberculous function, so eating crab is quite beneficial to the patients recovering from tuberculosis.

Removing blood stasis: Crab's functions include clearing heat and detoxifying the body, invigorating blood circulation and dredging collaterals, treating yin deficiency and nourishing the stomach, and crab provides dietary therapy for diseases such as blood stasis, injury, jaundice, ache in the waist and legs and rheumatic arthritis, etc.

Points of Attention for Different People

Suitable for elderly people: Crab's functions include strengthening bones and marrow, nourishing muscles and tendons, invigorating blood circulation, and relaxing main and collateral channels, and it provides dietary therapy for elderly people with aches in the waist and legs and rheumatic arthritis.

Suitable for patients with edema: The crab's functions include conserving strength, tonifying qi and easing swelling.

Not suitable for pregnant women: The crab claw is the coldest part of the crab, and it induces spontaneous abortion.

Food Compatibility and Incompatibility

Suitable: crab + asparagus = strengthens bones and teeth

Suitable: crab + bean curd = produces a restoring and anti-aging effect

Suitable: crab + green peppers = balances nutrition and helps digestion

Avoid: crab + tea leaves = slows down peristalsis and causes constipation

Avoid: crab + oysters = causes the rise of cholesterol

Cooking Tip

The living environment of the crab isn't clean, and its food carries pathogenic microorganisms such as bacteria, viruses and parasites, so it should be thoroughly washed before cooking, and do not eat dead or half-cooked crab.

Healthy Recipe

Crab and Beef Soup

Ingredients: 200 g (7 oz) beef; 80 g (3 oz) crabmeat; 200 g (7 oz) ox bone stew; 2 g (0.1 oz) each starch, monosodium glutamate, soy sauce, ginger powder, salt and sesame oil; 20 g (1 oz) water

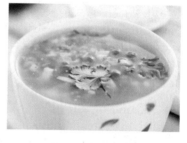

Preparation: ❶Wash and mince the beef, then add water, soy sauce, ginger powder and starch and mix it up; wash the crab meat and put it aside. ❷Put ox bone stew into the stockpot and bring it to a boil, then add beef to the soup and return to a boil. ❸Add the crabmeat to the soup and boil it for about three minutes; add salt and monosodium glutamate and sprinkle with sesame oil.

Sea Cucumber

Properties and taste: warm; salty
Channels of entry: heart, kidney
Essentials of pharmacopoeia: As recorded in the *Compendium of Materia Medica*, the sea cucumber nourishes the blood and cures recurrent dysentery.

Health Effects

Nourishing and building up the body: Sea cucumbers are high in protein and low in fat and cholesterol; they are tender and digestible, so they are an ideal food for elderly people and those with weak physiques.

Preventing anemia: The sea cucumber is rich in microelement iron, and it helps promote the circulation of iron in the blood, enhance hematopoietic functions and prevent anemia.

Tonifying the kidney and strengthening yang: The functions of sea cucumbers include tonifying kidneys and strengthening essence, tonifying yang and moistening dryness, and they can be used to treat consumptive diseases due to internal heat and yin deficiency, weakness, erectile dysfunction, spermatorrhea, premature ejaculation and frequent urination, etc.

Points of Attention for Different People

Suitable for elderly people: Sea cucumbers delay the senescence of muscles and enhance the body's immunity.

Suitable for patients with anemia: They are rich in iron and enrich the blood.

Suitable for men: The functions of sea cucumbers include tonifying the kidneys and benefiting essence, and they produce a good curative effect on erectile dysfunction and spermatorrhea.

Not suitable for patients with acute enteritis: The sea cucumber tends to cause diarrhea.

Food Compatibility and Incompatibility

Suitable: sea cucumbers + mutton = body building and energy replenishing

Suitable: sea cucumbers + black fungus = good for muscles and bones and promotes defecation

Avoid: sea cucumbers + persimmons = causes stomachache, nausea and vomiting

Cooking Tip

It is suggested that the water-swollen sea cucumber be cooked in a pot made of stainless steel or ceramic. Make sure that the vessels in contact with the sea cucumber including cookware, chopsticks and scissors, are free of greasy dirt.

Healthy Recipe
Sea Cucumber, Bamboo Fungus
and White Fungus Soup
Ingredients: 50 g (2 oz) sea
cucumber, 20 g (1 oz) each red
dates and white fungus, 10 g
(0.4 oz) each bamboo fungus and
Chinese wolfberries, 3 g (0.1 oz)
salt, 300 g (11 oz) water

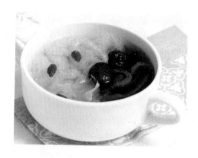

Preparation: ❶Soak sea cucumber and bamboo fungus in clean
water until they are well-swollen, wash and shred them; core and wash
the red dates and soak them for a few minutes; soak white fungus in
water until it is well-swollen, remove stems, wash and tear fungus into
small pieces. ❷Put white fungus and sea cucumber shreds into a pot of
water and bring to a boil over high heat. When the soup boils, adjust
the heat to low and boil for about 20 minutes; add Chinese wolfberries,
red dates and bamboo fungus shreds to the soup and boil for about 10
minutes; finish the soup by seasoning it with salt.

Shrimp

Properties and taste: warm;
sweet
Channels of entry: spleen,
kidney
Essentials of pharmacopoeia:
As recorded in the *Compendium
of Materia Medica*, shrimp soup can
be used to treat enclosed masses, expel smallpox and stimulate
the secretion of mother's milk; shrimp juice can be used to treat
wind phlegm; shrimp can be used to treat subcutaneous ulcers
if it is ground to cream.

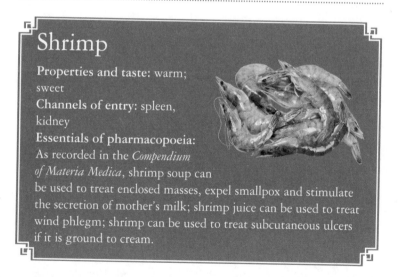

Health Effects
Protecting blood vessel: Shrimp is rich in magnesium, which helps
reduce the content of cholesterol in the blood, prevent arteriosclerosis

and expand the coronary arteries, and it can be used to prevent and cure hypertension and myocardial infarction.

Preventing osteoporosis: The shrimp shell is rich in calcium and chitin, and frequent consumption prevents osteoporosis.

Treating yin deficiency to tonify the spleen: The shrimp's functions include tonifying the kidneys and yang, treating yin deficiency to tonify the spleen, and it has a curative effect on erectile dysfunction caused by the deficiency of the kidneys and lack of appetite caused by the insufficiency of the spleen.

Improving eyesight and building up the body: The shrimp is rich in vitamin A, which protects eyes; it contains B vitamins, which eliminate fatigue and enhance physical strength.

Points of Attention for Different People

Suitable for beauty pursuers: Frequent shrimp intake nourishes the blood, moisturizes the skin, and enhances and brightens the complexion.

Suitable for men: The shrimp produces a good preventive effect on those with erectile dysfunction caused by the deficiency of the kidneys, premature ejaculation and spermatorrhea, soreness and weakness of the waist and knees and the weakness of limbs.

Not suitable for patients with skin disease: The shrimp belongs to stimulating food and it isn't suggested for these people.

Food Compatibility and Incompatibility

Suitable: shrimp + pumpkins = prevents black spots and wrinkles

Suitable: shrimp + tomatoes = improves heart and liver functions

Suitable: shrimp + papayas = helps the absorption of protein

Avoid: shrimp + persimmons = reduces protein absorption

Avoid: shrimp + fruit juice = causes abdominal distension and stomachache

Cooking Tip

The veins of shrimps are their digestive tracts, and there is excrement inside; the shrimp tastes like mud if the veins aren't removed, so remove them before cooking. Do not eat spoiled shrimp, and shrimp that are red and soft and without heads are not fresh, so do not eat them.

Healthy Recipe
Shrimp Soup

Ingredients: 200 g (7 oz) prawns;
100 g (3.5 oz) each cooked pork
tripe and squid; 50 g (2 oz)
crabsticks; 20 g (2 oz) rapeseed
greens; 5 g (0.2 oz) each salt, white
sugar and scallion oil; 200 g (7 oz)
fish soup

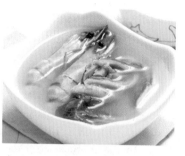

Preparation: ❶Devein, wash and scald the prawns; wash and
scald the rapeseed greens, soak them in cold water and remove
them; shred the cooked pork tripe; wash and shred the squid; cut the
crabsticks into strips. ❷Pour fish soup into the pot and add prawns,
pork tripe strips, squid and crabsticks to the soup, and boil it for about
three minutes; skim off the scum, add rapeseed greens to the soup and
boil it until it is cooked; season with salt and white sugar, and sprinkle
with scallion oil.

Clam

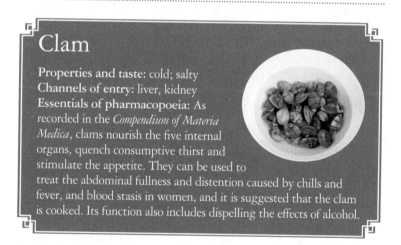

Properties and taste: cold; salty
Channels of entry: liver, kidney
Essentials of pharmacopoeia: As
recorded in the *Compendium of Materia
Medica*, clams nourish the five internal
organs, quench consumptive thirst and
stimulate the appetite. They can be used to
treat the abdominal fullness and distention caused by chills and
fever, and blood stasis in women, and it is suggested that the clam
is cooked. Its function also includes dispelling the effects of alcohol.

Health Effects

Preventing the chronic illnesses of old age: Clams are rich in
protein, fat, carbohydrates and all kinds of mineral substances,
vitamins, amino acids and taurine, etc., and they are an ideal food for
the chronic illnesses of old age.

Preventing a variety of diseases: The functions of clams include treating yin deficiency to moisten dryness, providing diuresis to subside swelling, and softening and resolving hard masses; clams also provide adjuvant therapy to diseases such as diabetes and dietary therapy for thyroid enlargement, jaundice, urinary retention and abdominal distension, etc.

Points of Attention for Different People

Suitable for patients with high cholesterol and hyperlipemia: Clam meat has the function of reducing cholesterol.

Suitable for patients with thyroid enlargement and bronchitis: The functions of clam meat include treating yin deficiency to improve eyesight, softening hard masses and removing phlegm.

Not suitable for people with deficiency-cold in the spleen and stomach: Clams are cold in properties, and excessive intake is not suggested for these people.

Food Compatibility and Incompatibility

Suitable: clams + ginger = produces an antipyretic and sterilization effect

Suitable: clams + spinach = improves anemia and promotes physical growth

Suitable: clams + carrots = protects eyes and enhances eyesight

Avoid: clams + oysters = destroys the absorption of iron

Cooking Tip

Seafood is rich in protein, and it spoils easily; therefore, before cooking it, trim and clean it thoroughly. When cooking clams, they should be heated at least for four minutes; or else they cause seafood poisoning and symptoms such as vomiting and diarrhea.

Healthy Recipe
Clams and Steamed Egg Soup

Ingredients: One egg, 200 g (7 oz) clams, 50 g (2 oz) straw mushrooms, 15 g (0.5 oz) shelled ginkgoes, 5 g (0.1 oz) salt, 1 g (0.04 oz) monosodium glutamate, 100 g (3.5 oz) each soup-stock and sesame oil, 30 g (1 oz) water

Preparation: ❶Wash ginkgoes and straw mushrooms, and dice straw mushrooms; soak the clams to let them spit out the sand. ❷Break the egg and put it into a steaming bowl; add a little salt and

water to it and stir it well; add
ginkgoes, straw mushrooms and
clams to it; put it into a steamer
and steam it with medium to low
heat for about 10 minutes and
then remove from the steamer.
❸Put soup-stock, salt and
monosodium glutamate into a pan

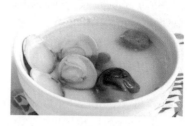

and bring to a boil, then sprinkle it with sesame oil and pour it into
the bowl loaded with steamed egg.

Kelp

Properties and taste: cold; salty
Channels of entry: stomach,
liver, kidney
Essentials of pharmacopoeia:
As recorded in the *Compendium
of Materia Medica*, kelp can be
used to treat thyroid enlargement
and scrofula.

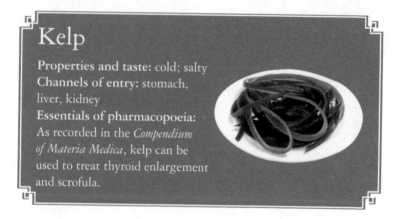

Health Effects

Supplementing iodine and preventing disease: Iodine is essential
for thyroid hormone synthesis, and people will catch "big neck"
disease if they lack iodine. Kelp is an ideal food for people with thyroid
hypofunction.

Reducing blood pressure and blood fat: Kelp is rich in
unsaturated fatty acid and dietary fiber, and it clears the cholesterol
sticking to the vascular walls and promotes the excretion of cholesterol;
the calcium it contains reduces the body's cholesterol absorption and
reduces blood pressure.

Expelling toxins and keeping people healthy: Kelp is rich in
iodine, and it is measured that every 100 grams of commercially available
dry kelp contains 0.7 to 0.8 milligrams; when the iodine is absorbed by
the human body, it promotes the excretion of hazardous substances.

Points of Attention for Different People

Suitable for patients with hyperplasia of the mammary glands: The iodine in kelp removes the risks of hyperplasia of the mammary glands.

Suitable for patients with hypertension: Kelp is rich in unsaturated fatty acid and dietary fiber, and it promotes the excretion of cholesterol.

Not suitable for pregnant women and parturients: The iodine in kelp may cause the developmental disorder of thyroxine of the fetus or infant.

Food Compatibility and Incompatibility

Suitable: kelp + bean curd = reduces blood pressure and prevents constipation

Suitable: kelp + white gourd = produces diuretic effect and eases swelling

Avoid: kelp + tea = affects the absorption rate of iron and calcium

Avoid: kelp + spinach = tends to cause lithiasis in the human body

Cooking Tip

Due to the water contamination that can be observed all around the world, there are some poisonous substances in kelp, so it is suggested to soak it for two to three hours before cooking. Change the water at least twice while soaking it, but do not soak it for more than six hours in case there is excessive loss of water-soluble nutrients.

Healthy Recipe
Spicy and Hot Kelp

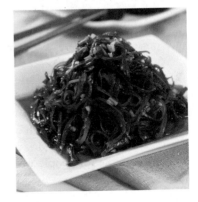

Ingredients: 300 g (11 oz) water-swollen kelp; 2 g (0.1 oz) each minced coriander, minced garlic, salt, monosodium glutamate, zanthoxylum oil, chili oil and sesame oil

Preparation: ❶Wash and shred the kelp and boil it for 10 minutes; remove it from water and cool; drain it well. ❷Dish up the shredded kelp, and season it with minced coriander, minced garlic, salt, monosodium glutamate, zanthoxylum oil, chili oil and sesame oil.

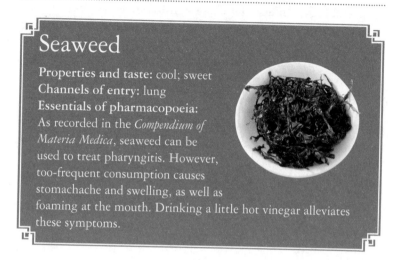

Seaweed

Properties and taste: cool; sweet
Channels of entry: lung
Essentials of pharmacopoeia:
As recorded in the *Compendium of Materia Medica*, seaweed can be used to treat pharyngitis. However, too-frequent consumption causes stomachache and swelling, as well as foaming at the mouth. Drinking a little hot vinegar alleviates these symptoms.

Health Effects

Enriching the blood and supplementing calcium: Seaweed is rich in elements such as calcium, phosphorus and iron; it is not only an ideal food in treating anemia in women and children, but it also promotes children's bone and tooth development.

Providing a diuretic effect and eliminating edema: Seaweed contains certain amount of mannitol, a natural diuretic, and it can help cure edema. Seaweed can also be used as adjuvant therapy to treat thyroid enlargement, scrofula and beriberi.

Expelling toxins: Seaweed is rich in iodine, and it promotes the excretion of hazardous substances and inflammation effusion.

Points of Attention for Different People

Suitable for children: Seaweed is rich in calcium, and it promotes children's bone and tooth development.

Suitable for patients with edema: The mannitol in seaweed has functions such as diuresis and easing swelling, etc.

Not suitable for people with weakness of the spleen and the stomach: It tends to cause diarrhea.

Food Compatibility and Incompatibility
Suitable: seaweed + honey = good for the health of the lungs and bronchia
   Suitable: seaweed + cuttlefish = improves complexion and aids body building
   Suitable: seaweed + eggs = promotes the absorption of calcium
   Avoid: seaweed + persimmons = affects calcium absorption rate
   Avoid: seaweed + vegetables with leaves of dark colors = tends to cause lithiasis

Cooking Tip
It is suggested that seaweed be soaked in water until it is well-swollen, and the water should be changed once or twice to clean the dirt in case it causes harm to the human body.

Healthy Recipe
Soybean Sprouts and Seaweed Soup

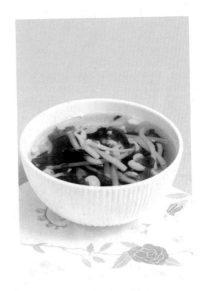

Ingredients: 150 g (5 oz) soybean sprouts, 10 g (0.4 oz) seaweed, 5 g (0.2 oz) minced garlic, 3 g (0.1 oz) salt, 4 g (0.1 oz) sesame oil, 2 g (0.1 oz) monosodium glutamate, 300 g (11 oz) water

   Preparation: ❶Soak the seaweed in water until it is well-swollen, wash it and tear it into small pieces; peel and wash the soybean sprouts. ❷Add the soybean sprouts and water to a pot and bring to a boil over high heat; adjust the heat to low and stew for 15 minutes. ❸Add seaweed, minced garlic, salt, monosodium glutamate and sesame oil to it and mix it up.

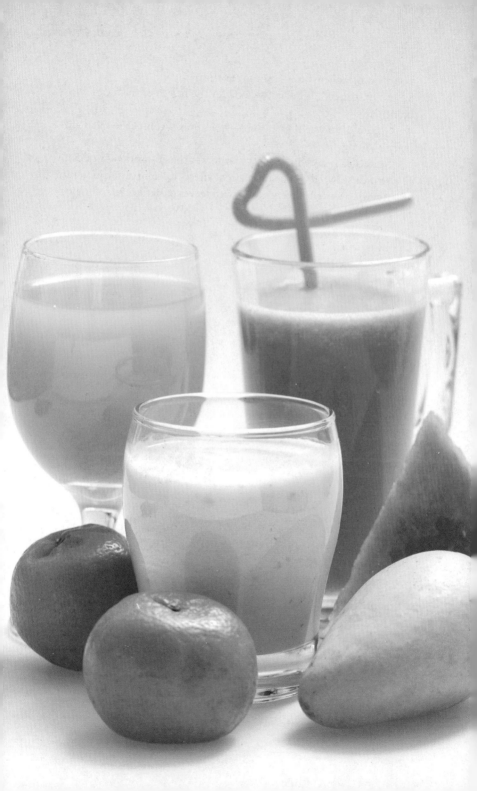

Chapter Seven

Drinks

Milk, soy milk, black tea and green tea are drinks familiar to people. Milk supplements calcium, soy milk delays senescence, black tea warms the stomach and green tea can help the body resist the radiation produced by electronics. Their health efficacy should not be underestimated. Why not enjoy your life by preparing a glass of soy milk or brewing a cup of black tea?

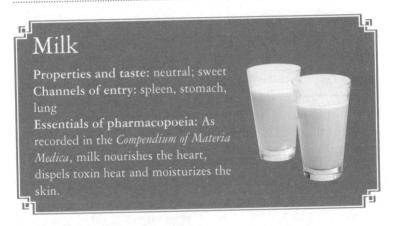

Milk

Properties and taste: neutral; sweet
Channels of entry: spleen, stomach, lung
Essentials of pharmacopoeia: As recorded in the *Compendium of Materia Medica*, milk nourishes the heart, dispels toxin heat and moisturizes the skin.

Health Effects

Preventing cardia-cerebrovascular disease: A variety of mineral substances in milk such as phosphorus, potassium and magnesium are quite balanced, and frequent milk consumption relieves hypertension and reduces the morbidity of cerebrovascular disease.

Promoting sleep: The milk contains L-tryptophan, which promotes sleep, and drinking milk before bed can improve sleep quality.

Calcium supplementation: It prevents osteoporosis if women frequently drink milk during pregnancy and menopause.

Protecting the skin: Milk is rich in vitamin A, which prevents dry and dark skin.

Points of Attention for Different People

Suitable for beauty pursuers: Milk contains iron, copper and vitamin A, which make skin smooth and moist.

Suitable for infants: Milk contains phosphorus, which promotes brain development in infants.

Suitable for pregnant women: Milk supplements calcium and promotes skeletal development of the fetus.

Suitable for elderly people: Milk is rich in mineral substances, and it prevents osteoporosis and cardiovascular and cerebrovascular diseases.

Food Compatibility and Incompatibility

Suitable: milk + honey = enhances immunity

Suitable: milk + papayas = improves complexion and protects skin

Avoid: milk + chives = reduces calcium absorption

Avoid: milk + sour juice = reduces the nutritive value

Eating Tip

Do not drink milk on an empty stomach—it is suggested that people eat some food before drinking milk to reduce the lactose concentration and promote nutrient absorption. Do not eat food that contains oxalic acid when drinking milk, in case it affects the body's calcium absorption. And it is not suggested that people heat milk with cookware made of copper, as it will destroy the milk's nutrients.

Healthy Recipes

Milk and Oat Porridge

Ingredients: 250 g (9 oz) milk, 50 g (2 oz) oatmeal, 10 g (0.4 oz) white sugar, 300 g (11 oz) water

Preparation: ❶Soak the oatmeal in clean water for 30 minutes. ❷Bring water to a boil over high heat, then add the oatmeal and boil it until it is cooked; turn off the stove. ❸Add

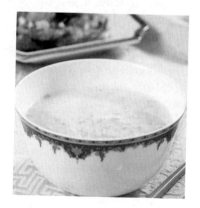

some milk and mix it evenly; stir
some white sugar into it and mix
it evenly.

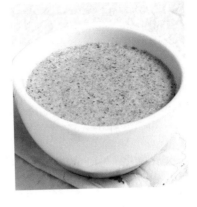

Vegetable and Milk Soup
Ingredients: 50 g (2 oz) each
broccoli and mustard leaves,
200 g (7 oz) milk, 3 g (0.1 oz)
white sugar

 Preparation: ❶Wash and
dice broccoli and mustard leaves;
put them into the juicer and
collect the vegetable juice. ❷Mix the milk with the vegetable juice,
pour it into a clean pot, boil it and stir some white sugar into it.

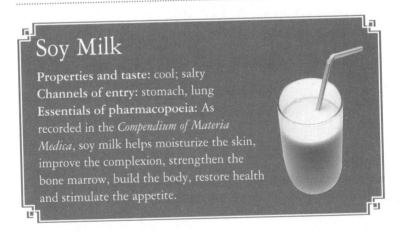

Soy Milk

Properties and taste: cool; salty
Channels of entry: stomach, lung
Essentials of pharmacopoeia: As
recorded in the *Compendium of Materia
Medica*, soy milk helps moisturize the skin,
improve the complexion, strengthen the
bone marrow, build the body, restore health
and stimulate the appetite.

Health Effects
Expelling toxins and nourishing the skin: Soy milk is rich in dietary
fiber, which reduces the time that toxins from food residue stay in the
human body, and it also reduces pimples and acne, and brightens and
improves the complexion.

 Weight loss and diuresis: Soy milk is rich in unsaturated fatty
acid, which decomposes the cholesterol in the human body, promotes
lipid metabolism, produces weight loss and has an anti-obesity effect.

Preventing cardiovascular disease: The functions of soy milk include restoring health and moistening dryness, clearing away the lung-heat to remove phlegm, promoting perspiration and diuresis; nutritionists consider it an ideal food for preventing and curing diseases such as hypertension, hyperlipidemia and atherosclerosis, etc.

Points of Attention for Different People
Suitable for elderly people: Frequent soy milk consumption prevents senile dementia.

Suitable for menopausal women: Soy milk regulates internal secretions, alleviates and improves climacteric symptoms and delays senescence.

Not suitable for patients with gastropathy: Bean products stimulate the secretion of gastric acid, worsen the condition and cause flatulence.

Food Compatibility and Incompatibility
Suitable: soy milk + cauliflower = improves complexion and aids skincare

Suitable: soy milk + pears = eliminates fatigue and enhances physical strength

Suitable: soy milk + milk = provides balanced nutrition

Avoid: soy milk + brown sugar = causes sedimentation and destroys nutrients

Eating Tip
Do not drink uncooked soy milk because it contains hazardous substances such as saponin and trypsin inhibitor, and it may cause poisoning symptoms such as nausea, vomiting and diarrhea if drunk without thorough cooking.

Healthy Recipes
Soy Milk
Ingredients: 80 g (3 oz) soybeans, 15 g (0.5 oz) white sugar (optional)

Preparation: ❶Soak soybeans in clean water for 10 to 12 hours and wash it. ❷Put the

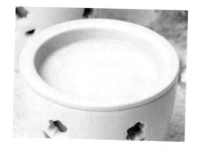

soaked soybeans into an automatic soy milk maker and feed water into it until the water is between the upper and the lower water lines; dish it up when the soy milk maker indicates that it is done. ❸Sieve it and season it with some white sugar according to personal preference.

Braised Vegetables with Soy Milk

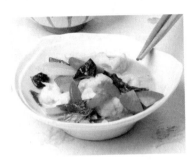

Ingredients: 500 ml (17 oz) soy milk, 100 g (3.5 oz) each cauliflower and rapeseed greens, 25 g (1 oz) fresh mushrooms and 50 g (2 oz) carrots, 2 g (0.1 oz) each salt and chopped scallions, 1 g (0.04 oz) monosodium glutamate, 100 g (3.5 oz) water

Preparation: ❶Trim and wash the cauliflower and break it into small pieces; trim, wash and halve the rapeseed greens; trim and wash the mushrooms, scald them in boiling water and then remove them; wash and dice the carrots. ❷Heat the oil in a pan, add chopped scallions and stir-fry until it smells delicious; put the carrot slices into the pan and stir-fry evenly; pour the soy milk and water and into the pan, and wait until it boils over high heat. ❸Put cauliflower and rapeseed greens into the pan and boil them for a few minutes; add the mushrooms, and season the dish with salt and monosodium glutamate.

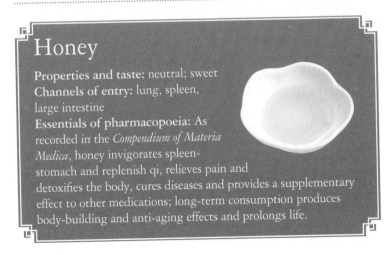

Honey

Properties and taste: neutral; sweet
Channels of entry: lung, spleen, large intestine
Essentials of pharmacopoeia: As recorded in the *Compendium of Materia Medica*, honey invigorates spleen-stomach and replenish qi, relieves pain and detoxifies the body, cures diseases and provides a supplementary effect to other medications; long-term consumption produces body-building and anti-aging effects and prolongs life.

Health Effects

Relieving pressure and improving sleep quality: Honey contains glucose, vitamins, magnesium, phosphorus, calcium and so on, so it helps regulate the nervous system, relieve stress and promote sleep.

Enhancing immunity: Honey provides quick energy replenishment, relieves tension and stress and enhances the resistance of the human body against diseases.

Treating skin injury: Bacteria cannot grow if honey is applied to a wound, and it helps cure moderate skin injuries, especially those from scalding.

Moisturizing the skin and moistening dryness: The functions of honey include moisturizing and nourishing the skin, making skin fine, smooth and supple.

Points of Attention for Different People

Suitable for beauty pursuers: Applying fresh honey to the skin provides moisturizing and nourishing effects and makes skin fine and smooth.

Suitable for people with insomnia: Drinking a spoonful of honey stirred into a glass of warm water before bed is an effective sleep aid.

Not suitable for patients with diabetes: Honey is high in sugar and calories.

Food Compatibility and Incompatibility

Suitable: honey + snow pears = relieves parched mouth and scorched throat

Suitable: honey + milk = clears internal heat and purges pathogenic fire

Suitable: honey + hawthorn berries = invigorates blood circulation and produce an anti-hypertensive effect

Eating Tip

Do not brew honey with boiling water. Honey is rich in enzymes, vitamins and mineral substances, and its natural color, flavor and taste will be lost and its nutrient content destroyed if it is brewed with boiling water. It is suggested that honey be brewed with warm water not exceeding 35 degrees Celsius (95 degrees Fahrenheit).

Healthy Recipes

Honeydew Sweet Lotus Root

Ingredients: 400 g (14 oz) lotus roots, 150 g (5 oz) glutinous rice, 150 g (5 oz) white sugar, three tablespoons of honey, 30 g (1 oz) sweet osmanthus, 100 g (3.5 oz) water

Preparation: ❶Peel and wash the lotus roots, cut off one end of roots and drain well. ❷Wash the glutinous rice and soak it for about four hours; mix it with white sugar evenly and

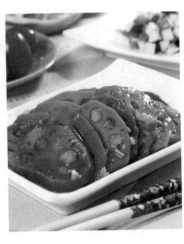

fill the holes of the lotus roots with the glutinous rice, put back the ends of the lotus roots that you cut off and fix them with toothpicks. ❸Lay the lotus roots on the steaming tray and steam for about one hour, then remove it and let it cool; remove the toothpicks and one end of lotus roots, and cut the lotus roots into slices about 1 cm thick. ❹Add water, white sugar and sweet osmanthus to the pot, skim off the foam and put the lotus root slices into the pot; boil over medium heat until the sugar juice becomes thick; put it aside until it is not hot and stir some honey into it.

Honey and Rapeseed Greens Juice

Ingredients: 50 g (2 oz) rapeseed greens, 80 g (3 oz) white radishes, 150 ml (5 oz) milk, 3 g (0.1 oz) honey

Preparation: ❶Wash rapeseed greens and white radishes and cut them into small strips. ❷Put the sliced ingredients and the milk into the automatic soy milk maker and press the "fruit and vegetable juice" button; after mixing it up, pour the fruit and vegetable juice into a glass and stir some honey into it.

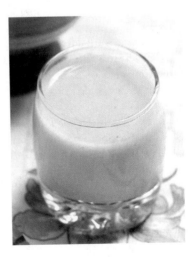

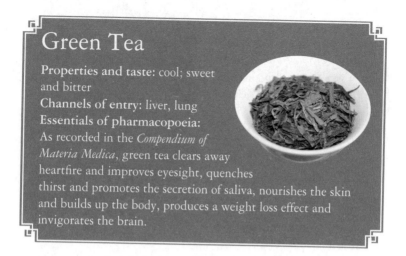

Green Tea

Properties and taste: cool; sweet and bitter
Channels of entry: liver, lung
Essentials of pharmacopoeia: As recorded in the *Compendium of Materia Medica*, green tea clears away heartfire and improves eyesight, quenches thirst and promotes the secretion of saliva, nourishes the skin and builds up the body, produces a weight loss effect and invigorates the brain.

Health Effects

Preventing diseases and providing a sterilizing effect: The catechinic acid in green tea produces an inhibiting effect on the pathogenic bacteria in the human body.

Preventing cardiovascular and cerebrovascular diseases: Frequent green tea consumption reduces blood glucose, blood lipids and blood pressure, and prevents cardiovascular and cerebrovascular diseases.

Preventing dental decay and clearing ozostomia: The catechinic acid in green tea inhibits caries-inducing bacteria and reduces the risks of dental plaque and periodontitis; it contains tannins, which provides a bactericidal effect, and effectively prevents ozostomia.

Preventing and treating cancer: Green tea produces an inhibiting effect on some cancers, and the catechinic acid it contains reduces the morbidity of skin cancer.

Points of Attention for Different People

Suitable for obese people: Green tea contains theophylline and caffeine, which reduce the accumulation of adipocyte.

Suitable for patients with heart disease: Green tea contains tannin, which delays the aging of the somatic system, as well as prevent and cure heart disease and stroke.

Not suitable for people with hypoglycemia: Green tea can reduce blood glucose in a short time, so it isn't suggested these people drink too much green tea.

Food Compatibility and Incompatibility

Suitable: green tea + longan = enriches the blood and clears heat

Suitable: green tea + watermelon = promotes body fluid production and quenches thirst

Avoid: green tea + rice wine = overburdens the heart

Eating Tip

Do not brew green tea for too long , or else the taste of the tea will be spoiled.

Healthy Recipes

Green Tea and Soy Milk with Jasmine Fragrance

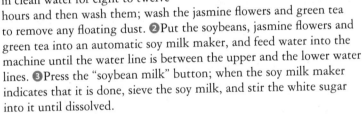

Ingredients: 60 g (2 oz) soybeans, 10 g (0.4 oz) each jasmine flowers and green tea, 10 g (0.4 oz) white sugar (optional)

Preparation: ❶Soak soybeans in clean water for eight to twelve hours and then wash them; wash the jasmine flowers and green tea to remove any floating dust. ❷Put the soybeans, jasmine flowers and green tea into an automatic soy milk maker, and feed water into the machine until the water line is between the upper and the lower water lines. ❸Press the "soybean milk" button; when the soy milk maker indicates that it is done, sieve the soy milk, and stir the white sugar into it until dissolved.

Green Tea, Lily Bulb and Soy Milk

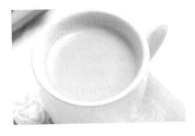

Ingredients: 50 g (2 oz) soybeans, 20 g (0.7 oz) mung beans, 10 g (0.4 oz) dried lily bulbs, 10 g (0.4 oz) crystal sugar (optional)

Preparation: ❶Soak soybeans and mung beans in clean water for eight to twelve hours and then wash them; wash away any floating dust from the green tea; wash the dried lily bulbs and soak them in water until they turn soft. ❷Put all the ingredients (except the crystal sugar) into an automatic soy milk maker, and feed water into it until the water is between the upper and the lower water lines; press the "soybean milk" button. When the soy milk maker indicates that the soy milk is done, sieve the soy milk, and stir crystal sugar into it until it is dissolved.

Black Tea

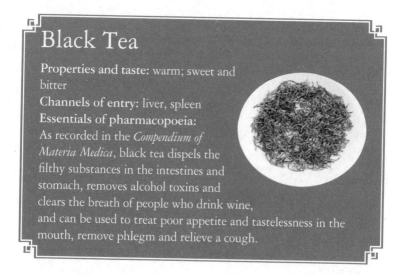

Properties and taste: warm; sweet and bitter

Channels of entry: liver, spleen

Essentials of pharmacopoeia:
As recorded in the *Compendium of Materia Medica*, black tea dispels the filthy substances in the intestines and stomach, removes alcohol toxins and clears the breath of people who drink wine, and can be used to treat poor appetite and tastelessness in the mouth, remove phlegm and relieve a cough.

Health Effects

Preventing myocardial infarction: Black tea is rich in the flavonoid compounds that remove free radicals and produce anti-acidification effects, and frequent consumption reduces the morbidity of myocardial infarction.

Providing anti-microbial effect and preventing cold: Black tea contains flavonoid compounds and has a sterilization function. It deprives the influenza virus of infectiousness, etc.

Nourishing and warming the stomach: The oxide that the black tea produces during the baking process promotes digestion and nourishes and warms the stomach.

Points of Attention for Different People

Suitable for women: It is suggested that women drink some black tea or brown sugar water before menstruation, as it helps eliminate cold syndrome and remove blood stasis.

Suitable for people with osteoporosis: A habit of drinking a small cup of black tea every day over years brings significant improvement for osteoporosis symptoms.

Suitable for patients with heart disease: Black tea improves the blood circulation of the coronary arteries and the heart's blood supply.

Food Compatibility and Incompatibility

Suitable: black tea + hawthorn berries = stimulates appetite to help digestion and produces blood-activating and stasis-dissolving effect

Suitable: black tea + milk = promotes digestion and eliminates fatigue

Suitable: black tea + ginger = protects and nourishes the skin

Avoid: black tea + spirits = harmful to the heart

Avoid: black tea + eggs = harmful to the digestion

Eating Tip

It is suggested that people drink black tea before the meal. Black tea is produced through fermentation and baking, and the tea polyphenol undergoes an enzymatic oxidation reaction, decreasing its oxidase content and thus decreasing its irritant effect on the stomach. Black tea does not impair the stomach; rather it nourishes the stomach.

Healthy Recipes

Black Tea and Rice Porridge

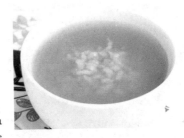

Ingredients: 100 g (3.5 oz) rice, 10 g (0.4 oz) black tea, 4 g (0.1 oz) salt, 500 g (18 oz) water

Preparation: ❶Wash and soak the rice for 30 minutes; wrap the tea leaves in a gauze. ❷Bring a pot of water to a boil, then put the tea bag in the pot; when the tea is thoroughly brewed and it gives off strong fragrance, remove the tea bag from the pot. ❸Put the rice into the tea and boil it over high heat; when it boils, adjust the heat to low and boil it until the rice is well-cooked and the porridge is quite thick, and season it with some salt.

Black Tea with Milk

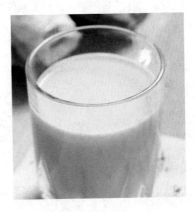

Ingredients: 5 g (0.2 oz) black tea, 200 ml (7 oz) fresh milk

Preparation: ❶Scald the teacup in boiling water and put the tea leaves in the teacup; pour 100 g (3.5 oz) boiling water of about 95 degrees Celsius (about 200 degrees Fahrenheit) into the teacup, brew the tea for 10 to 20 seconds and sieve it. ❷Stir the fresh milk into the tea.

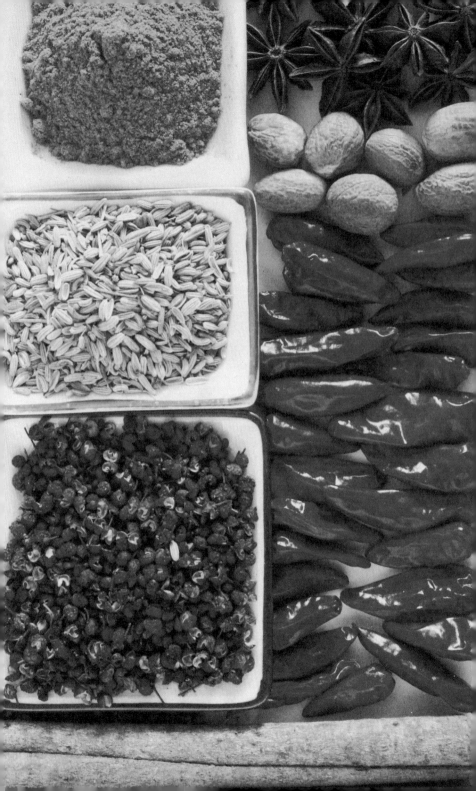

Chapter Eight
Seasonings

Seasonings are necessities in every meal, and they not only improve color, flavor and taste of dishes, but also whet the appetite. Their health-enhancing functions should not be overlooked. Seasonings not only improve the taste and flavor of a dish, but also keep people healthy if used properly.

Vinegar

Properties and taste: neutral; sour
Channels of entry: liver, stomach
Essentials of pharmacopoeia:
As recorded in the *Compendium of Materia Medica*, vinegar eliminates swollen abscesses, dispels dampness, gets rid of toxins and supplements other medications.

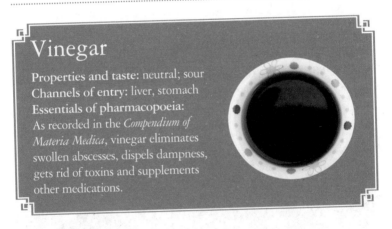

Health Effects

Sterilization and softening blood vessel: Vinegar has anti-bacterial properties and the ability to sterilize, and it effectively prevents intestinal problems, influenza and respiratory tract diseases; meanwhile, it helps soften blood vessels and reduce cholesterol, so it is an ideal food for the patient with cardia-cerebrovascular disease.

Whetting the appetite: Vinegar promotes the secretion of saliva and gastric juices, and it helps digestion, improves the appetite and relieves stasis.

Helping sleep: Vinegar eliminates fatigue and aids sleep, and it aids hair growth, improves the complexion, helps weight loss and acts as an antihypertensive.

Points of Attention for Different People

Suitable for people with dyspepsia: Vinegar whets the appetite and promotes secretion of digestive juices.

Suitable for patients with pharyngitis: Rinsing the mouth with vinegar can treat mild pharyngitis.

Not suitable for patients with osteoporosis: Vinegar softens the bones and causes decalcification, which destroys the dynamic equilibrium of human body and aggravates osteoporosis.

Not suitable for patients with stomach ulcers: Vinegar is rich in organic acid, which promotes the secretion of digestive juices, increases gastric acid and aggravates gastropathy.

Healthy Recipe

Mixed Endive with Vinegar

Ingredients: 200 g (7 oz) endive; 50 g (2 oz) deep-fried peanuts; 2 g (0.1 oz) each mature vinegar, minced garlic, white sugar, salt, monosodium glutamate and sesame oil

Preparation: ❶Remove the stem from the endive, wash and drain it well. ❷Mix all the seasonings to prepare a sauce; put the endive and fried peanuts into a container, season them with the sauce, mix them evenly, and dish it up.

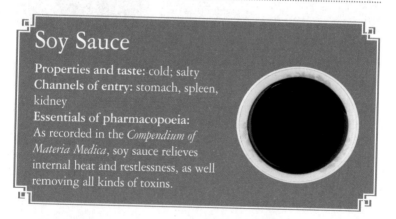

Soy Sauce

Properties and taste: cold; salty
Channels of entry: stomach, spleen, kidney
Essentials of pharmacopoeia:
As recorded in the *Compendium of Materia Medica*, soy sauce relieves internal heat and restlessness, as well removing all kinds of toxins.

Health Effects

Improving the flavor of dish and stimulating the appetite: Soy sauce improves the flavor and appearance of food and whets appetite. Adding it after the dish is cooked preserves the soy sauce's effective amino acid and nutrient content.

Preventing cardiovascular disease: Soy sauce contains phytoestrogens, which reduce cholesterol and reduces the morbidity of cardiovascular disease. Soy sauce also produces a natural antioxidant component, which helps reduce the damage that free radicals cause to the human body.

Points of Attention for Different People

Suitable for most people: Soy sauce improves tastes, flavor and appearance of food, as well as offering supplemental nutrients.

Not suitable for patients with gastropathy: Soy sauce is acidic in nature and excessive consumption causes hyperacidity.

Healthy Recipe
Sauced Beef

Ingredients: 500 g (18 oz) silverside beef; 50 g (2 oz) large-fruited Chinese hawthorn berries; 10 g (0.4 oz) ginger slices; 20 g (0.7 oz) scallion strips; 10 Sichuan peppers; one aniseed; 2 g (0.1 oz) each fennel, cassia bark, salt and white sugar; 50 ml (2 oz) soy sauce

Preparation: ❶Wash the silverside and cut off the fascia along its veins, then cube it; wash and put aside the large-fruited Chinese hawthorn berries. ❷Put diced beef, hawthorn berries, scallion strips and ginger slices into 500 g (18 oz) clean water. When it boils, add soy sauce, white sugar, Sichuan peppers, aniseed, fennel and cassia bark to the water and boil them for about 20 minutes. ❸Adjust the heat to low and boil it for about two hours; add some salt, simmer the soup until it thickens and remove the beef; when the beef becomes cool, cut it into thin slices to serve.

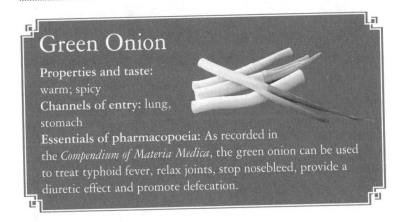

Green Onion

Properties and taste: warm; spicy

Channels of entry: lung, stomach

Essentials of pharmacopoeia: As recorded in the *Compendium of Materia Medica*, the green onion can be used to treat typhoid fever, relax joints, stop nosebleed, provide a diuretic effect and promote defecation.

Health Effects

Sterilization and curing the cold: Green onions contain volatile oil and capsaicin that give off a pungent smell, and they have strong bactericidal effect. The volatile oil and the capsaicin slightly stimulate the relevant glands when they are released, which induces perspiration, eliminates phlegm and provides a diuretic effect. Therefore, the green onion can be used to cure a cold.

Refreshing the mind: Green onions stimulate the secretion of gastric juices and whet the appetite. If people eat green onion with food rich in vitamin B_1, it produces a refreshing effect.

Points of Attention for Different People

Suitable for people with loss of appetite: Green onions stimulate the body's secretion of digestive juices, tonifying the spleen and stimulating and improving the appetite.

Suitable for cancer patients: The pectin in green onions produces anti-cancer effects, and the allicin in green onions also inhibits the growth of cancer cells.

Not suitable for patients with bromhidrosis: Green onions are quite irritative to the sweat glands. People should be cautious in eating green onions in the summer.

Healthy Recipe

Green Onion Stalk Porridge

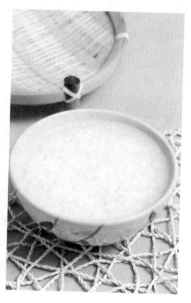

Ingredients: 50 g (2 oz) rice, 10 g (0.4 oz) white stalk of green onion, 2 g (0.1 oz) salt, 500 g (18 oz) water

Preparation: ❶Wash and soak the rice for 30 minutes; wash and cut the green onion stalk into strips. ❷Turn on the stove and place the pot on it. Pour some boiling water into the pot and add the rice to the water; when the rice is almost cooked, add the strips of green onion stalk to the pot; when the rice is well-cooked, season the porridge with some salt.

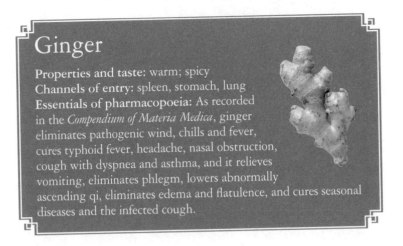

Ginger

Properties and taste: warm; spicy
Channels of entry: spleen, stomach, lung
Essentials of pharmacopoeia: As recorded in the *Compendium of Materia Medica*, ginger eliminates pathogenic wind, chills and fever, cures typhoid fever, headache, nasal obstruction, cough with dyspnea and asthma, and it relieves vomiting, eliminates phlegm, lowers abnormally ascending qi, eliminates edema and flatulence, and cures seasonal diseases and the infected cough.

Health Effects

Stimulating the appetite and promoting digestive functions: The gingerol in ginger stimulates the gustatory nerves on the tongue and the receptors on the gastric mucosa, stimulating appetite and tonifying the spleen, promoting digestion function and whetting the appetite.

Sterilization and curing diseases: The volatile oil in ginger provides sterilization effects, and adding some ginger to a dish not only improves the flavor but also removes toxins from the food. Drinking ginger soup when you have a cold also produces good preventive and curative effects.

Points of Attention for Different People

Suitable for people with carsickness and seasickness: Ginger produces a good curative effect on nausea and vomiting.

Not suitable for patients with skin diseases: Ginger is a pungent and stimulating food, and it will aggravate gargalesthesia and other symptoms if a patient eats too much of it.

Not suitable for patients with hemorrhoids: Ginger is quite irritating, and it produces internal heat, so it aggravates the symptoms of hemorrhoids.

Healthy Recipe

Brown Sugar and Ginger Soup

Ingredients: 150 g (5 oz) ginger, 5 g (0.2 oz) brown sugar, 500 g (18 oz) water

Preparation: ❶ Wash the ginger and smash it without peeling it. ❷ Put the ginger and brown sugar into a pot and add water; when it boils over high heat, adjust the heat to low and continue to boil for another 45 minutes.

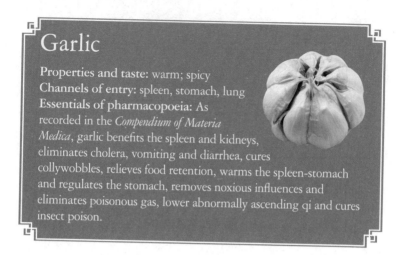

Garlic

Properties and taste: warm; spicy
Channels of entry: spleen, stomach, lung
Essentials of pharmacopoeia: As recorded in the *Compendium of Materia Medica*, garlic benefits the spleen and kidneys, eliminates cholera, vomiting and diarrhea, cures collywobbles, relieves food retention, warms the spleen-stomach and regulates the stomach, removes noxious influences and eliminates poisonous gas, lower abnormally ascending qi and cures insect poison.

Health Effects

A strong sterilization effect: The capsaicin in garlic has strong sterilizing capability, and frequent garlic consumption prevents influenza and wound infection, cures infectious diseases and expels parasites.

Preventing cancer and tumor: The germanium and selenium in garlic inhibit the growth of tumor and cancer cells. American researchers believe that garlic has more anticancer potential than any other food in the world.

Points of Attention for Different People

Suitable for patients with diabetes: Garlic is rich in selenium, and it has certain effect on the synthesis of insulin.

Not suitable for patients with stomach ulcers: Garlic is irritating to the gastric mucosa.

Healthy Recipe

Garlic Porridge

Ingredients: One bulb of garlic; 100 g (3.5 oz) rice; 10 g (0.4 oz) Chinese wolfberries; 2 g (0.1 oz) each sesame oil, salt and monosodium glutamate; 500 g (18 oz) water

Preparation: ❶Peel and crush the garlic; wash and soak the rice for 30 minutes. ❷Put the rice and water into a pot, and bring to a boil over high heat. When the rice is cooked, add the garlic and Chinese wolfberries to the mixture and continue to boil it into porridge; season it with monosodium glutamate and salt and sprinkle it with sesame oil.

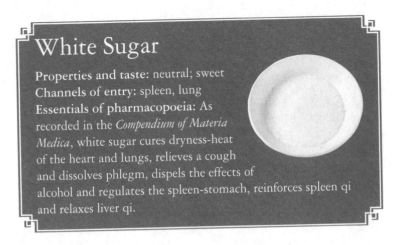

White Sugar

Properties and taste: neutral; sweet
Channels of entry: spleen, lung
Essentials of pharmacopoeia: As recorded in the *Compendium of Materia Medica*, white sugar cures dryness-heat of the heart and lungs, relieves a cough and dissolves phlegm, dispels the effects of alcohol and regulates the spleen-stomach, reinforces spleen qi and relaxes liver qi.

Health Effects

Clearing internal heat and diminishing inflammation: According to modern research, white sugar changes the acid-base property of wounds, promotes the growth of histocyte and accelerates wound healing.

Moistening the lung and promoting body fluid secretion: The functions of white sugar include regulating the spleen-stomach and benefiting the spleen, moistening the lungs to treat yin deficiency and relieving the cough, and if eaten properly, white sugar helps the body absorb calcium.

Points of Attention for Different People

Suitable for people with lung deficiency and cough: White sugar moistens the lungs and promotes body fluid secretion, invigorates the stomach-spleen and alleviates acute diseases.

Suitable for patients with hypoglycemia: Eating white sugar relieves glucose deficiency.

Not suitable for patients with diabetes: It is a taboo for these patients.

Healthy Recipe
Preserved Tomatoes with Sugar

Ingredients: 400 g (14 oz) tomatoes; 2 g (0.1 oz) each white sugar, sesame oil and honey

Preparation: ❶Wash and dice the tomatoes, and dish them up. ❷Put honey and sesame oil into a bowl, mix them up; pour it in a dish and sprinkle with white sugar.

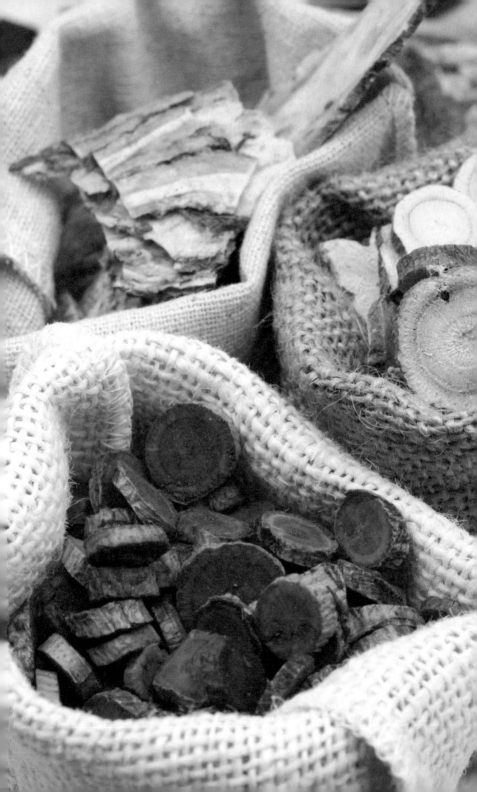

Chapter Nine

Nourishing
Traditional Chinese Medicines

Many traditional Chinese medicines are of both pharmaceutical and food resources, such as Chinese wolfberries, lotus seeds and lily bulbs. Food pairing and preparation are also important for these tonic medicines. With suitable cooking and eating methods, people can harness the health-enhancing benefits of these ingredients.

Codonopsis

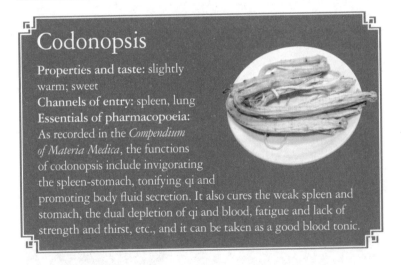

Properties and taste: slightly warm; sweet
Channels of entry: spleen, lung
Essentials of pharmacopoeia: As recorded in the *Compendium of Materia Medica*, the functions of codonopsis include invigorating the spleen-stomach, tonifying qi and promoting body fluid secretion. It also cures the weak spleen and stomach, the dual depletion of qi and blood, fatigue and lack of strength and thirst, etc., and it can be taken as a good blood tonic.

Health Effects

Improving immunity: Codonopsis is an important medicine that benefits qi and tonifies the spleen, and it contains saponin, synanthrin, micro-alkaloid and starch, etc., which provide various tonifying effects on different organs; it also helps boost immunity.

Benefiting qi and nourishing blood: Codonopsis not only benefits qi but also enriches the blood, and frequent consumption is quite good for the people with pale complexion, feebleness and dizziness.

Points of Attention for Different People

Suitable for people with dyspepsia: Codonopsis is an important medicine for invigorating the spleen and tonifying qi, and it corrects gastrointestinal dysfunction and promotes digestion.

Suitable for people with anemia: Codonopsis enhances hematopoietic functions.

Not suitable for people with insomnia: Codonopsis excites the nervous system and aggravates the symptoms of insomnia.

Healthy Recipe

Stewed Sea Cucumbers with Codonopsis and Chinese Wolfberries

Ingredients: 300 g (18 oz) water-swollen sea cucumbers; 10 g (0.4 oz) each codonopsis and Chinese wolfberries; 2 g (0.1 oz) each vegetable oil, scallion strips, soy sauce, rice wine, salt and water starch

Preparation: ❶Dice the sea cucumbers, quick-boil them and remove from water, and let them dry in the air; slice the codonopsis, wash the Chinese wolfberries, and put them into a small bowl loaded with some water; steam them until they are cooked. ❷Pour some oil into the pan and add the scallion strips to it; fry them until fragrant; put the sea cucumber into the pan, and add rice wine, salt and soy sauce to it and stir-fry it for a moment. Put the steamed codonopsis and Chinese wolfberries together with the soup into the pan and thicken them with mixture of cornstarch and water.

Chinese Wolfberry (Goji Berry)

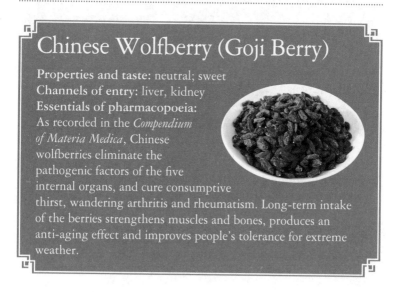

Properties and taste: neutral; sweet
Channels of entry: liver, kidney
Essentials of pharmacopoeia:
As recorded in the *Compendium of Materia Medica*, Chinese wolfberries eliminate the pathogenic factors of the five internal organs, and cure consumptive thirst, wandering arthritis and rheumatism. Long-term intake of the berries strengthens muscles and bones, produces an anti-aging effect and improves people's tolerance for extreme weather.

Health Effects

Nourishing the eyes and improving eyesight: Chinese wolfberries are rich in carotene, vitamin A, vitamin B_1, vitamin B_2, vitamin C, calcium, iron and more, and all of them are essential nutrients to keep eyes healthy. Because the berry has good nourishing effects on the eyes, it is commonly known as the "eyes protector."

Anti-cancer and preventing "three highs": The functions of the Chinese wolfberry include relieving high blood pressure, high blood lipids and high blood glucose, and it prevents atherosclerosis, protects the liver, reduces the risk of fatty liver and promotes hepatocyte regeneration, and it also has an anti-cancer effect.

Points of Attention for Different People

Suitable for computer users: Chinese wolfberries contain essential nutrients for the eyes and can relieve eyestrain.

Suitable for patients with fatty liver: Chinese Wolfberries to some extent inhibits the accumulation of fat in the hepatocyte and promotes hepatocyte regeneration.

Not suitable for people with fever: Chinese wolfberries are a tonic and aggravate the symptoms.

Healthy Recipe

Spinach and Chinese Wolfberries Porridge

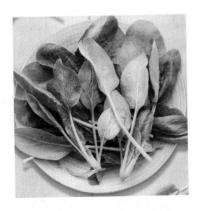

Ingredients: 100 g (3.5 oz) each spinach and millet, 15 g (0.5 oz) Chinese wolfberries, 500 g (18 oz) water

Preparation: ❶Trim and wash the spinach, scald it and remove from water, then cut it into small strips; wash the millet and Chinese wolfberries. ❷Turn on the stove and place an earthen pot on it. Pour 500 g water into the earthen pot and bring it to a boil; add the millet and return to a boil over high heat. ❸When it boils, adjust the heat to low and boil for 15 minutes; add the Chinese wolfberries and boil until the millet is well-cooked; put the spinach strips into the casserole and mix it evenly; cook until the porridge boils.

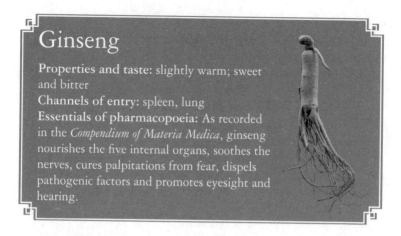

Ginseng

Properties and taste: slightly warm; sweet and bitter

Channels of entry: spleen, lung

Essentials of pharmacopoeia: As recorded in the *Compendium of Materia Medica*, ginseng nourishes the five internal organs, soothes the nerves, cures palpitations from fear, dispels pathogenic factors and promotes eyesight and hearing.

Health Effects

Benefiting qi: Ginseng is known as the "king of herbs," and its functions include benefiting qi, tonifying the spleen and benefiting the lungs, promoting body fluid secretion and quenching thirst, soothing the nerves and improving brain health, and it is also known as a "qi benefiting panacea."

Anti-aging: Ginseng contains more than ten varieties of ginsenoside, and it also contains saccharides, a variety of amino acids and vitamins, and its functions include delaying cell senescence and prolonging the life of cells, thus providing an anti-aging effect.

Points of Attention for Different People

Suitable for people with hypoimmunity: Ginseng enhances the body's resistance against harmful factors.

Suitable for people with anemia: Ginseng produces protective and stimulating effects on the hematopoietic function of marrows and helps relieve anemia.

Not suitable for patients with insomnia: Ginseng excites the nervous centralis, so it will aggravate insomnia.

Healthy Recipe

Ginseng and Poria Cocos Porridge

Ingredients: 3 g (0.1 oz) ginseng; 15 g (0.5 oz) each Poria cocos, millet and rice; 30 g (1 oz) yam; 500g (18 oz) water

Preparation: ❶Wash ginseng, Poria cocos and yam, and bake them; grind them into fine powder and put aside; wash millet and rice. ❷Put millet and rice into a pottery pot and pour 500 g water into the pot; bring it to a boil over high heat, then add the ground powder and some water to it; stew it over low heat until the porridge is cooked.

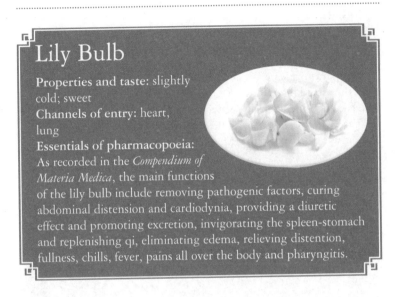

Lily Bulb

Properties and taste: slightly cold; sweet
Channels of entry: heart, lung
Essentials of pharmacopoeia: As recorded in the *Compendium of Materia Medica*, the main functions of the lily bulb include removing pathogenic factors, curing abdominal distension and cardiodynia, providing a diuretic effect and promoting excretion, invigorating the spleen-stomach and replenishing qi, eliminating edema, relieving distention, fullness, chills, fever, pains all over the body and pharyngitis.

Health Effects

Nourishing the heart and moistening dryness: The lily bulb's functions include calming the heart and soothing the nerves, clearing heat and cooling the blood, and they can be used to cure diseases such as fever after recovering from heat illness, absent-mindedness, insomnia and dreaminess. The fresh lily bulb is rich in plant mucilage, and it moistens dryness and clears heat, and it is also used to cure a cough caused by lung dryness and lung heat.

Building up the body and nourishing the skin: The lily bulb is rich in protein, saccharides, starch and mineral substances, and it builds the body and strengthens the bones; the mucilage and vitamins it contains are beneficial to the metabolism of dermal cells, and frequent consumption provides skin protection and nourishing effects.

Points of Attention for Different People

Suitable for the cancer patients: The functions of lily bulbs include improving immunity and inhibiting the proliferation of cancer cells.

Suitable for people with insomnia: Lily bulbs contain a special glycoside, which has a sedative and hypnotic effect.

Not suitable for people with diarrhea: Lily bulbs are slightly cold in properties and can aggravate the symptoms.

Healthy Recipe
Lily Bulbs and Asparagus Soup
Ingredients: 50 g (2 oz) fresh lily bulbs, 100 g (3.5 oz) asparagus, 5 g (0.2 oz) salt, 2 g (0.1 oz) monosodium glutamate
Preparation: ❶Wash and break the lily bulbs into small pieces; wash the asparagus and cut it into strips. ❷Bring a pot of water to a boil, then add the lily bulb sections to the pot and boil them until they are 70 percent cooked. ❸Add the asparagus strips to the soup and boil until they are cooked; season the soup with salt and monosodium glutamate.

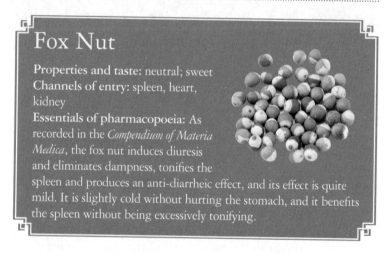

Fox Nut

Properties and taste: neutral; sweet
Channels of entry: spleen, heart, kidney
Essentials of pharmacopoeia: As recorded in the *Compendium of Materia Medica*, the fox nut induces diuresis and eliminates dampness, tonifies the spleen and produces an anti-diarrheic effect, and its effect is quite mild. It is slightly cold without hurting the stomach, and it benefits the spleen without being excessively tonifying.

Health Effects
Reinforcing the kidney and arresting seminal emission: The fox nut contains starch, fat, calcium, phosphorus, iron, riboflavin, vitamin C and so on, and it is a good medicine that has functions such as nourishment, body building, tonifying the spleen, curing diarrhea, invigorating the kidneys and controlling nocturnal emissions.

Fighting cancer: The fox nut strengthens the small intestine's absorption function and raises the concentration of carotene in the blood, reducing the probability of lung cancer and gastric cancer.

Points of Attention for Different People

Suitable for people with deficiency of the kidney: The functions of fox nut include nourishment, body building, tonifying the spleen, curing diarrhea and supplementing the kidneys to control nocturnal emissions.

Not suitable for people with constipation: The fox nut produces a potent astringency-inducing effect.

Healthy Recipe
Yam and Fox Nuts Porridge

Ingredients: 50 g (2 oz) each common yam rhizome and fox nuts, 100 g (3.5 oz) rice, 2 g (0.1 oz) each vegetable oil and salt, 500 g (18 oz) water

Preparation: ❶Wash the rice, season it with a little salt and mix them up; bring a pot of water to a boil and add the rice. ❷Soak yam and fox nuts for a few minutes, remove impurities and wash them; dice the yam and put it aside. ❸When the rice boils, put yam and fox nuts into the pot and boil them; when the porridge is cooked, season it with vegetable oil and table salt.

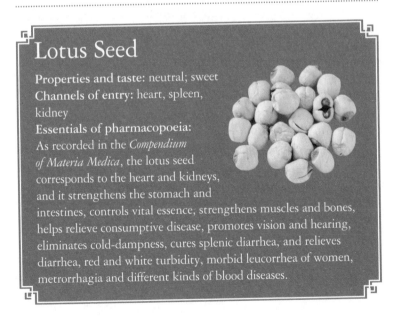

Lotus Seed

Properties and taste: neutral; sweet
Channels of entry: heart, spleen, kidney
Essentials of pharmacopoeia:
As recorded in the *Compendium of Materia Medica*, the lotus seed corresponds to the heart and kidneys, and it strengthens the stomach and intestines, controls vital essence, strengthens muscles and bones, helps relieve consumptive disease, promotes vision and hearing, eliminates cold-dampness, cures splenic diarrhea, and relieves diarrhea, red and white turbidity, morbid leucorrhea of women, metrorrhagia and different kinds of blood diseases.

Health Effects

Balancing acid-base: The lotus seed is rich in calcium, and it strengthens tendons and bones, soothes the nerves and nourishes the heart. It promotes the three major metabolism systems of the human body, that is, protein, fat and saccharides, and it maintains the body's acid-base equilibrium.

Clearing internal heat and hemostasis: The green and tender germ inside the lotus seed is called the lotus plumule. Lotus plumules are bitter in taste and cold in properties, and their functions include clearing away the heart fire and removing heat, hemostasis and arresting seminal emission, and they cure diseases such as insomnia, restlessness, hematemesis and spermatorrhea caused by heart fire hyperactivity.

Points of Attention for Different People

Suitable for people with insomnia: The lotus seed nourishes the heart, soothes the nerves and eliminates fatigue.

Suitable for the weak patients recovering from diseases: The lotus seed has good nourishing effects on people with macronosia, postpartum women and elderly people with a weak physique.

Not suitable for people with constipation: The lotus seed does not digest easily, and it would aggravate the symptoms.

Healthy Recipe

Hawthorn Berries, Red Dates and Lotus Seeds Porridge

Ingredients: 100 g (3.5 oz) rice, 50 g (2 oz) hawthorn berries, 30 g (1 oz) each red dates and lotus seeds, 10 g (0.4 oz) brown sugar, 500 g (18 oz) water

Preparation: ❶Wash and soak the rice for 30 minutes; wash the red dates and lotus seeds; core the red dates and remove the lotus plumules. ❷Pour water into the pot, add rice, red dates and lotus seeds and boil them; when the lotus seeds are thoroughly cooked, put the hawthorn berries into the pot, boil it until it becomes porridge; stir some brown sugar into the porridge.